Types of Tea and Their Health Benefits
By Angela Jewitt

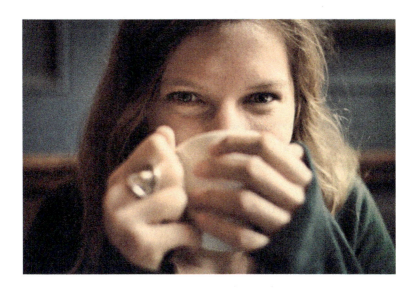

Including History, Types of Tea, Health Benefits, Side Effects, Uses and Flavours.

Copyright and disclaimer

The information in this book is not intended as a substitute for the medical advice of doctors and physicians. The reader should regularly consult a doctor or physician in matters relating to his/her health and particularly with respect to any symptoms that may require diagnosis or medical attention.

Published by
WHYTBANK PUBLISHING, TD1 1UF, UK

ALL RIGHTS RESERVED.

This book contains material protected under international and federal copyright laws and treaties.
Any unauthorised reprint or use of this material is strictly prohibited.
No part of this book may be reproduced or transmitted in any form or by any means, electronic, mechanical or information storage and retrieval system without express written permission from the author.

Copyrighted © 2015

ISBN: 978-0-9930278-2-6

Forward

Second to water, tea is the most highly consumed beverage in the world. But what makes it so popular? Tea has a naturally bitter flavour, depending on the type of plant it is steeped from, and it has a unique aroma. Most importantly, however, tea can provide a wide variety of health benefits including, perhaps, a reduced risk for cancer and enhanced protection from other degenerative diseases. If you are curious to learn more about tea including its history, preparation, and different types, this book is the perfect place for you to start.

Acknowledgements

I would like to extend my deepest gratitude to my family who supported me as I pursued this project. Special thanks to my friends who helped me to assemble and taste such a wide variety of different teas in the name of research.

Table of Contents

Chapter One: Introduction _____ 1

Chapter Two: The History of Tea _____ 3

    1.) The Discovery of Tea _____ 4

    2.) Expansion of Tea to Europe _____ 6

    3.) History of Tea in Britain _____ 8

    4.) Modern Day Tea Drinking _____ 11

Chapter Three: How to Prepare Tea _____ 14

    1.) Tips for Tea Preparation _____ 15

    2.) Utensils and Equipment for Brewing Tea _____ 18

    3.) Methods for Brewing Tea _____ 22

        a.) Instructions for Tea Preparation _____ 24

        b.) Preparation Tips for Types of Tea _____ 29

    4.) Making Homemade Tea Bags _____ 33

Chapter Four: Health Benefits of Tea _____ 36

    1.) Top 10 Health Benefits of Tea _____ 37

    2.) Tea Benefits for Weight Loss _____ 39

    3.) Tea Benefits for Inflammation _____ 40

    4.) Tea Benefits for Mental Health _____ 42

    5.) Tea Benefits for Diabetes _____ 44

    6.) Tea Benefits for Heart Health _____ 45

    7.) Tea Health Benefits Chart _____ 47

Chapter Five: Types of Tea _____ 49

    a.) Green Tea _____ 50

        Jasmine Tea _____ 53

- Lonjing _____ 54
- Matcha _____ 54
- Sencha _____ 55
- b.) Black Tea _____ 56
  - Assam _____ 60
  - Almond Tea _____ 61
  - Darjeeling _____ 61
  - Ceylon _____ 61
  - Masala Tea _____ 62
- c.) White Tea _____ 63
- d.) Oolong Tea _____ 65
- e.) Herbal Tea _____ 68
  - Barley Tea _____ 71
  - Catnip Tea _____ 71
  - Calendula Tea _____ 71
  - Chaga Tea _____ 72
  - Chamomile Tea _____ 73
  - Cinnamon Tea _____ 73
  - Coca Tea _____ 74
  - Comfrey Tea _____ 74
  - Corn Silk Tea _____ 74
  - Damiana Tea _____ 75
  - Echinacea Tea _____ 75
  - Dandelion Tea _____ 75
  - Fennel Tea _____ 76
  - Fenugreek Tea _____ 77
  - Ginger Tea _____ 77
  - Gingko Biloba Tea _____ 78
  - Ginseng Tea _____ 78
  - Graviola Tea _____ 79
  - Holy Basil Tea _____ 79
  - Honeybush Tea _____ 79
  - Hibiscus Tea _____ 79
  - Horsetail Tea _____ 80
  - Kava Tea _____ 81
  - Lemon Balm Tea _____ 81

Licorice Tea	82
Mint Tea	82
Moringa Tea	82
Mother's Milk Tea	83
Mulberry Tea	83
Mullein Tea	83
Nettle Tea	84
Parsley Tea	84
Poppy Seed Tea	85
Raspberry Tea	86
Red Bush Tea	86
Red Clover Tea	86
Rooibos Tea	87
Rosehip Tea	87
Saffron Tea	87
Sage Tea	88
Senna Tea	88
Sassafras Tea	89
Tulsi Tea	89
Turmeric Tea	90
Yarrow Tea	90
f.) Floral/Fruit Tea	92
Apple Tea	94
Black Currant Tea	94
Blueberry Tea	94
Chrysanthemum Tea	95
Cranberry Tea	95
Lavender Tea	95
Linden Tea	96
Peach Tea	97
Pineapple Tea	97
Rose Tea	97
Vanilla Tea	98
Chapter Six: Where to Buy Tea	**99**
1.) Tips for Buying Tea Online	**100**

- **2. Recommended Online Suppliers** **102**
  - a.) Verdant Tea 103
  - b.) Crimson Lotus Tea 103
  - c.) In Pursuit of Tea 103
  - d.) Red Blossom Tea Company 104
  - e.) Rishi 104
  - a.) Nothing But Tea 105
  - b.) Mad Hatter Tea 105
  - c.) Jenier World of Teas 105
  - d.) Tea Palace 106
  - e.) Drury Tea and Coffee Company 106
- **3.) Finding a Local Tea Shop** **107**

Conclusion *109*

References *110*

Image Credits *114*

Index *118*

Chapter One: Introduction

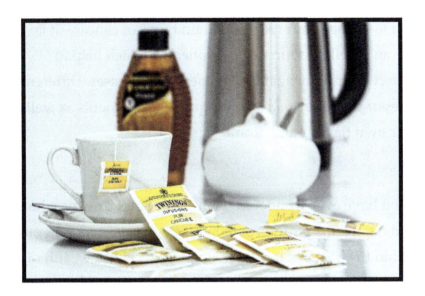

Tea is a delicious beverage, often served hot, that is made by steeping the leaves of certain species of plant in hot water. Second to water, tea is the most highly consumed beverage in the world and it has been enjoyed by humans for many centuries. Though real tea is made from the leaves of the *Camellia sinensis* plant, so-called "herbal" teas can be made from an infusion of certain herbs or fruit. Some examples of herbal tea include rosehip tee, rooibos tea, and chamomile tea.

Chapter One: Introduction

Not only does tea have a unique flavour but it is known around the world for providing a wide variety of health benefits. Tea contains valuable antioxidants which may help to reduce your risk for certain types of cancer – it is also an excellent source of polyphenols which help to protect your body against degenerative diseases. Different types of tea have their own unique sets of benefits as well as their own flavour and aroma.

If you have ever wondered where tea comes from or what kind of benefits it can provide, this book is perfect for you. Within the pages of this book you will receive a wealth of information about tea including its history, its side effects and benefits, its preparation, and the many different types of tea. By the time you finish this book you will have a firm understanding of not only where tea comes from and what it is, but you will have learnt which types of tea provide which benefits and what they taste like.

Chapter Two: The History of Tea

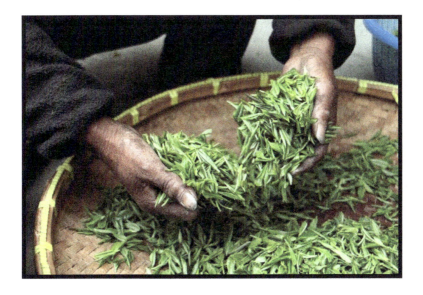

As you have already learned, tea is the most commonly consumed beverage in the world. Today there are hundreds of different types of tea, not to mention countless herbal teas made from plants besides the tea plant. Before you learn the benefits of this wonderful beverage and before we get into its preparation methods, it would be helpful for you to understand a little bit about the background and history for tea.

Chapter Two: The History of Tea

1.) The Discovery of Tea

Though the exact details for the discovery of tea are unknown, legend has it that tea was first discovered by the Emperor of China, Shen Nung, in 2737 BC. According to the legend, the Emperor was sitting under a tree while his servant boiled his drinking water. Some of the leaves from the tree blew into the pot of boiling water to create an infusion. As a renowned herbalist, Shen Nung was curious to see what this accidental concoction would taste like so he gave it a try. The tree under which the Emperor was sitting was a *Camellia sinensis* tree, the type of plant used to create most of the world's tea today.

It is impossible to know how true this story actually is but, regardless of its origins, tea became an important part of Chinese culture after its discovery. In fact, tea was popular in China for many centuries before it was even introduced to Western cultures. Containers used for storing tea have been found in ancient tombs in China dating as far back as the Han dynasty between 206 and 220 AD. Though the exact origins of tea are unknown, there is documentation to support the idea that tea became firmly established in China as its national beverage during the Tang dynasty which lasted from 618 to 906 AD.

Tea became such a popular drink in China that, during the late eighth century, the writer Lu Yu wrote an entire book about it. This book was called the Ch'a Ching, which translates to Tea Classic. Shortly after this book was released, tea was introduced in Japan by Japanese Buddhist monks who had spent time studying in China. Tea quickly became an important aspect of Japanese culture, just as it had in China. This fact is most strongly evidenced by the development of the Tea Ceremony. This ceremony was developed by Japanese monks as a means of sharing tea in a spiritual, sacred manner.

2.) Expansion of Tea to Europe

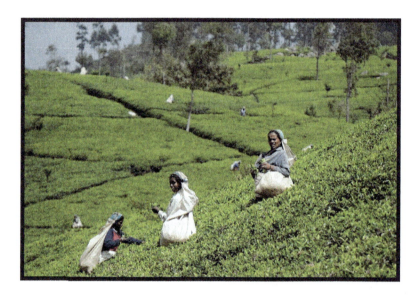

Again, the exact origins of tea in Europe are up for debate, but there are some mentions of tea in Europe beginning in the latter half of the sixteenth century. These records come from Portuguese traders and missionaries who were living in the East. Though some of these individuals may have brought samples of tea back to their home countries, the Portuguese were not the first to start shipping tea as a commercial import – it was the Dutch. At the end of the sixteenth century, the Dutch began to encroach on the trading routes used by the Portuguese in the East.

Chapter Two: The History of Tea

By the turn of the century, the Dutch had created a trading post on Java, an Indonesian island in the Indian Ocean. It was from this island that the first consignment of tea was sent in 1606 from China to Holland. After this first consignment, tea quickly became a very fashionable drink among Dutch citizens and it spread from there to other countries in Western Europe. For many years tea was an expensive drink and therefore only enjoyed by the rich.

Today, Britain is known for being a nation of tea drinkers – but they did not get that name overnight. It is likely that sailors manning the ships for the British East India Company brought some tea home from Asia as gifts, but the first dated reference to tea in Britain did not occur until 1658. This mention came in the form of an advertisement in the *Mercurius Politicus*, a London newspaper, in September of 1658. This advert announced that a beverage called "China Drink" was available for sale at a coffee house located in Sweeting's Rents in the city. The first coffee house in London had only been established in 1652, so tea was still largely unfamiliar when it appeared 6 years later.

Chapter Two: The History of Tea

3.) *History of Tea in Britain*

The turning point for tea in Britain came in the 1660s when King Charles II married Catherine of Braganza, a Portuguese princess and tea addict. It was Catherine's love of the drink that made it popular as a fashionable beverage at court. It quickly spread among the wealthy and eventually made its way into the lower classes as well. Samuel Pepys, a member of Parliament and English naval administrator, wrote in his diary on September 25, 1660, "I did send for a cup of tee (a China drink) of which I never had drank before." Four years later, in 1664, the East India Trading Company decided to capitalize on the popularity of tea in Britain and placed its first order for 100 lbs. (45.3 kg).

The spread of tea throughout Britain can largely be credited to the coffee houses that began to spring up all over the country. Coffee houses back then were used as much for relaxation and pleasure as they were as locations for business transactions. Men were the most frequent patrons of these coffee houses, though upper class women enjoyed the beverage in their own homes. For many years, tea was

Chapter Two: The History of Tea

still too expensive for the working class to enjoy – this was largely due to the system of taxation.

The first tax on tea was introduced in 1689 – it was so high, at 25p per pound, that it nearly stopped tea sales. In 1692 the tax was reduced to 5p, but the rate continued to change until 1964 when duties on tea were finally abolished. One of the most significant results of the taxation on tea was the development of smuggling and adulteration in the tea trade. By the 18th century tea had become extremely popular, but it was still too expensive for many Britons to enjoy.

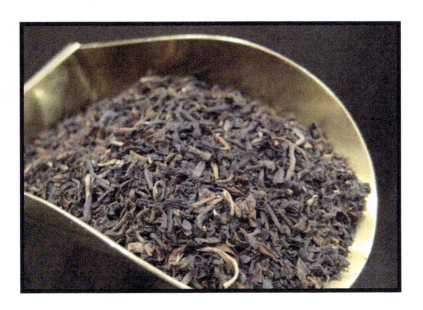

Chapter Two: The History of Tea

To capitalise on the popularity of this beverage, criminal gangs began to smuggle it into the country to avoid the taxes. This system began small with a few smugglers selling small quantities of tea to personal contacts but it quickly grew into a large network of organized crime which imported nearly 7 million pounds of tea per year – at this time legal imports totalled only 5 million pounds. Though smuggled tea was more affordable for working class citizens, its quality was much lower than legal imports because its quality was not controlled by customs.

Illegal tea imports were often mixed with the leaves of other plants – they were also mixed with leaves that had already been brewed and then dried. Due to this adulteration, the colour of illegal tea imports was not convincing. To solve this problem, smugglers sometimes added substances to the tea to correct the problem. These substances ranged from sheep's dung to poisonous copper carbonate. By 1784, the British government realised that taxation on tea was causing more problems than it was solving. It was then that British Prime Minister, William Pitt the Younger, reduced the tax on tea from 119% to 12.5%. When legal tea suddenly became affordable, smuggling halted almost immediately.

Chapter Two: The History of Tea

4. Modern Day Tea Drinking

During the 18th century the debate about tea taxation was incredibly prominent, but so was the debate regarding the health benefits of tea. At this time wealthy philanthropists worried that drinking tea in excess would lead to melancholy and weakness among the working classes. These effects were not of concern among the wealthy classes because work ethic and strength of labour were of much lower importance. The debate regarding the health benefits of tea continued into the 19th century until a new generation of philanthropists realised that tea was incredibly beneficial for the temperance movement. Tea was often offered at temperance meetings as an alternative to alcohol.

In 1834 the East India Trading Company's monopoly on trade with China ended. When the monopoly ended, the company started to think about growing tea in China. But because India had always been the centre of the company's operations, the company began to cultivate tea in India, starting in Assam. Though there were a few hiccups along the way, the first auction of Assam tea occurred in Britain in

Chapter Two: The History of Tea

1839. By 1888, British imports of tea from India were actually greater than they were from China.

By 1901, the annual consumption of tea had skyrocketed to more than 6 pounds per head – this was largely due to the availability of inexpensive imports from Sri Lanka and India. It was around this time that tea had finally become established as an integral part of British culture. When the First World War came about, the government took steps to oversee the importation of tea into the country to make sure that its morale-boosting benefits could be enjoyed by the lower classes at an affordable price. The British government again took control of imports during the Second World War, rationing tea from 1940 until 1952.

In 1952 the London Tea Auction returned – it had begun in 1706 and it was the centre of the world's tea industry. Not only did this auction improve the availability of tea, it also encouraged worldwide trade communication. The last tea auction was held on June 29, 1998. As the tea auction declined in importance, another aspect of tea drinking arose – the tea bag. Tea bags were first used in the United States during the early 20th century. It wasn't until the 1970s, however, that sales took off in Britain. Today, it is hard to imagine life without tea bags. Developments in modern science have also proved a link between drinking tea and several significant health benefits. For these reasons, tea will always remain a popular beverage.

Chapter Three: How to Prepare Tea

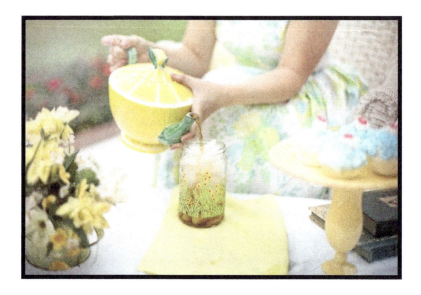

As you probably already know, there are a wide variety of different teas out there. Different types of tea can be prepared using different methods. Most people are familiar with tea bags which you simply steep in hot water, but fresh tea can also be made using dried tea leaves and other plant-based materials. In this chapter you will receive step-by-step instructions for several different preparation methods for tea.

Chapter Three: How to Prepare Tea

1.) Tips for Tea Preparation

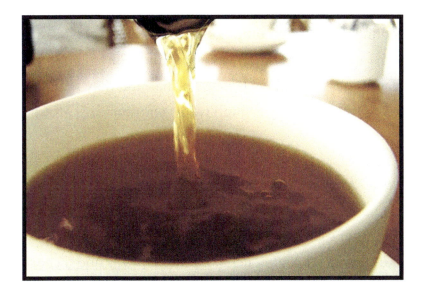

One of the best ways to prepare fresh tea is to use dried tea leaves and to steep them in hot water. There are several factors to consider when preparing green tea including the type of water, water temperature, steeping time, and the amount of tea leaves used. Changing any of these factors will result in a change of flavour and aroma for the tea.

Why is water temperature so important for brewing a quality cup of tea? The temperature of the water you use to steep tea has a direct effect on the aroma of the tea as well

Chapter Three: How to Prepare Tea

as its flavour. Different components of the tea dissolve at different temperatures. Temperatures above 175°F (80°C) will draw out the catechins, the astringent component of tea, while the flavour components (the amino acids) can be drawn out at lower temperatures around 122°F (20°C). Certain types of tea have strong aromas and they will only be brought out with very high water temperatures around 212°F (100°C).

To illustrate this concept, consider the example of several different types of green tea: sencha, high-grade sencha, gyokuro, bancha, and hojicha. <u>Below you will find a chart detailing the ideal water temperature and infusion time for each type of green tea:</u>

Type	Amount of Tea	Water Temperature	Infusion Time
Sencha	¾ tablespoon (2.0 grams)	175°-195°F (80° - 90°C)	60 seconds
Sencha (high-grade)	½ tablespoon (2.0 grams)	158°F (70°)	120 seconds
Gyokuro	1 tablespoon (3.3 grams)	140°F (60°C)	120 seconds
Gyokuro (high-grade)	1 tablespoons (3.3 grams)	122°F (50°C)	150 seconds

Chapter Three: How to Prepare Tea

Bancha	1 tablespoon (3.0 grams)	Boiling	30 seconds
Hojicha	1 tablespoon (3.0 grams)	Boiling	30 seconds

Given the table above, you can see how different types of tea require different water temperatures and infusion times. Standard gyokuro tea should be steeped at a fairly low temperature to draw out its flavour slowly while high-grade sencha should be steeped at a higher temperature to draw out the flavour while minimizing astringency. At temperatures around 175°F (80°C), the catechins in tea start to release, giving tea its characteristic bitter (astringent) flavour. It isn't until the higher temperatures around 200°F (100°C) that the full aroma of the tea comes out.

Chapter Three: How to Prepare Tea

2. Utensils and Equipment for Brewing Tea

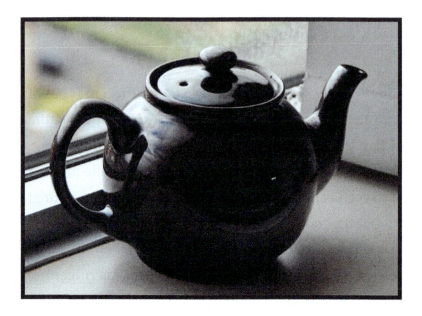

In order to be successful in any task, you need to have the proper tools and equipment on hand – it is no different with brewing tea. Different cultures use different utensils for brewing and serving tea, so the utensils required for a particular brewing method might vary depending on the type of tea you are preparing. The most common utensils and equipment needed to brew tea include the following:

- Teapot
- Tea cups

Chapter Three: How to Prepare Tea

- Tea caddy
- Tea scoop
- Tea infuser

Teapot

The teapot is the most important piece of equipment you will need to properly brew tea. Teapots can be made from a variety of materials including ceramic, glass, and metal. Teapots also come in a variety of sizes and shapes depending on the type of tea they are used to prepare – choosing the right teapot for a particular type of tea will help to bring out the tea's individual flavour and aroma. Some people recommend using different teapots for different teas because some strongly flavoured teas (like black tea) may season the teapot and it could affect the flavour if you use it for another type of tea.

When brewing high-grade teas like sencha and gyokuro, it is best to use a small teapot. Other teas, like hojicha and genmaicha, are best prepared in larger teapots. Many teapots feature a strainer at the bottom of the spout to catch the tea leaves as you pour the tea. If your teapot does not have this feature you will need to use some kind of insert to hold the tea leaves during the infusion period.

Chapter Three: How to Prepare Tea

Tea Cups

The second most important utensil you need to prepare and serve tea is, of course, your tea cups. Like teapots, tea cups vary greatly in size and shape. Small cups are often used for high-grade and strongly flavoured teas where the serving size is small. Larger tea cups may be used for mild teas and herbal teas. The type of tea cup you use to serve tea is largely a matter of preference, but certain cultures use special cups for certain types of tea. For example, Chinese black tea is typically served in very small ceramic cups.

Tea Caddy

Though this particular piece of equipment is not mandatory, it is highly recommended especially if you plan to use dried tea leaves. To keep your tea leaves fresh, you need to keep them from coming into contact with moisture or air. A tea caddy is simply a container used to store tea leaves and they can be made from a variety of materials, though metal is common. Japanese tea caddies typically have both an inner and an outer lid to ensure the maximum degree of air tightness. If you do not have a tea caddy you can use a glass jar or some other kind of airtight container that you have around the house.

Chapter Three: How to Prepare Tea

Tea Scoop

This utensil is what you use to measure your tea leaves when preparing fresh tea – it is how you transfer your tea leaves from the tea caddy to the teapot. Tea scoops are typically made from bamboo, wood, or metal and they come in a variety of shapes and sizes.

Tea Infuser

A tea infuser is simply a device used to contain loose tea leaves during steeping. Infusers come in a variety of shapes and sizes, some for infusing a single mug of tea and others for brewing a whole pot. Tea infusers are typically made from mesh or metal and they are perforated to allow the hot water to come into contact with the tea leaves.

Chapter Three: How to Prepare Tea

3. Methods for Brewing Tea

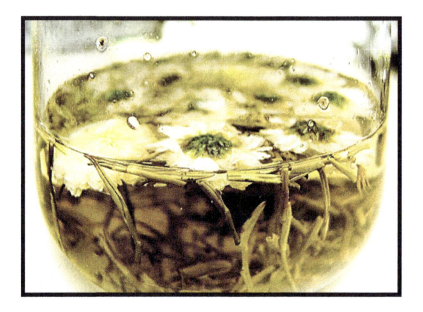

There are many different types of tea and each type of tea has its own unique brewing method. Each brewing method is designed to bring out the maximum flavour and aroma of the particular type of tea. <u>Some of the most common tea brewing methods are listed below</u>:

- Tea Bags
- Loose Leaf Tea
- Herbal Decoction
- Herbal Infusion

Chapter Three: How to Prepare Tea

- Herbal Water
- Gongfu

Before getting into the details of different tea preparation methods, there are a few things you need to know. First, it is important to use the best quality tea you can, no matter which type of tea you choose. Choosing a high-quality tea will ensure the maximum degree of flavour and aroma. Do not let high prices fool you or stop you from buying good quality tea. Even a tea that costs $100 per pound will only cost you about 50 cents per cup to prepare.

Another factor you need to consider is the water you use to prepare your tea. Always use fresh water from the tap or water that has been filtered – do not use water that has previously been boiled or that has been sitting tepid for a while. Next, use the right amount of tea. For most types of tea you will need about 1 rounded teaspoon of loose leaf tea per 8-ounce (240ml) cup. Certain teas are finer or denser than others, so pay attention to any special instructions that come with the tea when you buy it.

Chapter Three: How to Prepare Tea

You have already learned about the importance of using the right water temperature for steeping your tea but you also need to make sure you give the tea enough time to expand while it is steeping. If you are using an infuser, make sure there is room for the tea leaves to expand 3 to 5 times their size as they become saturated with water. Finally, once your tea has steeped for the desired amount of time, separate the leaves from the water to stop the steeping. If you keep the tea leaves in the water for too long, the tea will turn bitter.

a.) Instructions for Tea Preparation

Now that you know the basics about tea preparation you may be interested to learn about the different methods. In this section you will receive step-by-step instructions for the different methods used to prepare tea.

Tea Bags

Using tea bags is perhaps the easiest method of brewing tea and it is a great way to brew individual servings. To brew tea using tea bags, fill a kettle with tap water and bring it to a boil. Place your tea bag in a mug then pour in enough hot water to fill the mug. Let the tea steep for as long as desired – it will depend on the type of tea. Remove the tea bag and sweeten your tea if desired.

Loose Leaf Tea

There are several different ways you can brew loose leaf tea – it just depends on the type of equipment you have available. If you have a teapot that is equipped with a strainer, you can fill the teapot with water and then place the tea in the strainer. If your teapot does not have a strainer you will need to use an infuser. Infusers come in a variety of shapes and sizes, so choose one that fits your teapot and that can accommodate the amount of tea you want to prepare.

To brew tea using a teapot equipped with a strainer, add the desired amount of tea leaves directly to the teapot. Fill a kettle with water and heat it to the desired temperature (it will vary depending on the type of tea). Pour the hot water into the teapot and let it steep for the desired amount of time. Pour the tea into your cups and serve. To brew tea using an infuser you will follow the same steps but, instead of adding the tea leaves directly to the teapot, you'll place them in the infuser and then place the infuser in the teapot.

Herbal Decoction

An herbal decoction is a method for preparing herbal tea using dried herbs or other plant-based materials. To make an herbal decoction, place 2 to 8 teaspoons (10 to 40 grams) of the herb in a saucepan and add 4 cups (1000ml) of water. Let the herbs soak overnight then bring the mixture to a boil. Reduce the heat and simmer the mixture until it reduces to ¼ its original volume, about 1 cup (250ml). You can then strain the mixture to remove the dried herbs.

Herbal Infusion

An herbal infusion is very similar to an herbal decoction except that it does not involve heat. Simply place 2 to 4 teaspoons (10 to 20 grams) of the herb in a bowl and cover with 1 cup (250ml) of water. Let the mixture soak for at least 12 hours then strain it to remove the solids.

Herbal Water

Herbal water is very similar to both of the previous methods, herbal decoction and herbal infusion. The main

Chapter Three: How to Prepare Tea

difference is that the liquid is not reduced by evaporation. To make herbal water, the most basic form of herbal tea, simply combine 2 to 4 teaspoons (10 to 20 grams) with 1 cup (250ml) of water and boil until hot then strain the liquid. As an alternative you can simply add hot water to the herbs and infuse for the desired length of time.

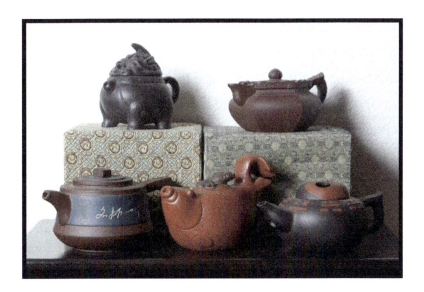

Gongfu

The gongfu method of preparing tea is the traditional Chinese way of making tea using a Yixing pot. A Yixing pot is a clay teapot and it has been used in China since the 15th century. This type of teapot is specifically meant for use

Chapter Three: How to Prepare Tea

with oolong and black teas, though they can be used with white and green tea if the water is allowed to cool before pouring it into the pot. To prepare tea using the gongfu method begin by heating your water in a kettle then pour it into the teapot to warm it. Next, pour the water into your tea cups to warm them then discard the water.

After warming the teapot and the cups, add the loose leaf tea to the pot and cover it with the lid. Let the tea warm for 10 to 20 seconds then remove the lid and fill the pot with water and cover it with the lid. Immediately pour the water into your cups then discard it again. Refill the pot with water and let the tea steep for 20 to 30 seconds, as desired. Pour the tea into tasting cups to serve.

Chapter Three: How to Prepare Tea

b.) Preparation Tips for Types of Tea

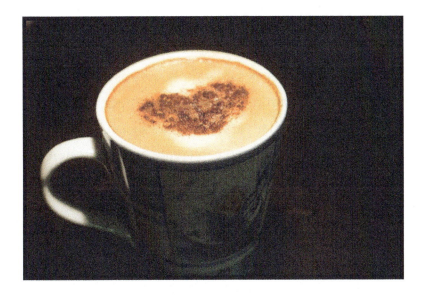

The preparation methods described in the last section can be used to brew most types of tea. There are certain types of tea, however, which require special preparation methods. These types of tea may include chai tea (Indian tea), dark tea, flowering tea, iced tea, and matcha tea. In this section you will receive step-by-step instructions for preparing these speciality teas.

Chapter Three: How to Prepare Tea

Chai Tea

The Indian word for tea is chai, so technically the term "chai tea" is redundant. The traditional Indian tea masala chai is made with black tea, milk, and sweetener as well as a unique blend of spices. Some of the spices used in chai include cinnamon, cardamom, nutmeg, ginger, cloves, and pepper. Recipes for chai vary from one region to another. To prepare chai at home you can create a concentrated chai mixture that you can add to freshly brewed black tea. To prepare this concentrated mixture combine 1 can of sweetened condensed milk with 1 tablespoon of chai spice blend and stir well. When you are ready to prepare your chai, steep 1 teaspoon of Indian black tea in 8 ounces (250ml) of hot water for 2 to 4 minutes. Strain to remove the tea leaves then stir in 1 tablespoon of your chai concentrate.

Dark Tea

Dark tea is a type of aged tea that comes from China. This tea has undergone a secondary fermentation process so it has a dark, early aroma with a floral flavour. To prepare dark tea you will need a little more leaf than you would with other teas – use one heaped teaspoon (about 5 grams) of tea per 8-ounce (250ml) cup. Steep the tea in 208° to 212°F

Chapter Three: How to Prepare Tea

(98° to 100°C) water for about 4 to 6 minutes. You can re-steep dark tea leaves several times, if you like.

Flowering Tea

This type of tea is also known as blooming tea, blossoming tea, or flower tea. Flowering teas consist of bundles of tea leaves that are gathered in balls or rosettes, often wrapped around a dried flower. When steeped in water, the bundle expands and "flowers," releasing the tea into the hot water. To prepare flowering tea, place the bundle in a glass teapot or mug. Heat your water to boiling then pour it gently over the bundle and let it steep for 3 to 4 minutes or until it has fully "bloomed".

Iced Tea (Hot Brew)

To make iced tea you can either use tea bags or loose leaf tea. The important thing to keep in mind with iced tea is that you need to brew it stronger than you normally would because it will be diluted when you add ice. To use loose leaf tea, use 1 teaspoon per 6 ounces of water. Bring your water to boil in a tea kettle then add about 8 to 10 teaspoons (40 to 50 grams) of loose tea per 4 cups (1000ml) water. Let the tea steep for 3 to 5 minutes then strain it and serve over

Chapter Three: How to Prepare Tea

ice. To use tea bags, steep 8 tea bags in 8 cups (2000ml) of hot water.

Iced Tea (Cold Brew)

To prepare cold brewed iced tea, place 8 to 10 teaspoons (40 to 50 grams) of loose tea in a gallon-sized (4.5 litre) jug. Fill the jug with cold water and then let it steep for at least 8 hours, or overnight. Strain the mixture to remove the lose tea and then serve over ice.

Matcha Tea

Matcha is a type of powdered green tea that it often used in Japanese tea ceremonies. This tea is produced using the highest grade available of Japanese gyokuro tea and it has a sweet, astringent flavour. To prepare matcha tea, scoop about ½ teaspoon (2.5 grams) of matcha powder into a tea bowl. Pour in ¼ cup (120ml) of simmering water then stir slowly until the powder is dissolved. Keep whisking the mixture until it is slightly foamy then enjoy hot.

Chapter Three: How to Prepare Tea

4. Making Homemade Tea Bags

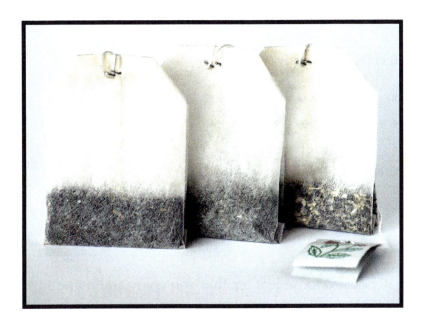

If you are looking for a quick and easy way to brew tea, tea bags are definitely the way to go. To use a tea bag, you simply place it in your mug and then fill the mug with hot water. The longer you let the tea bag steep, the stronger your tea will be. The downside of tea bags is that they are only available for certain types of tea. If you like the flavour of loose leaf teas or if you have a preference for a certain type of tea, you may be able to make your own tea bags at home by following the steps that are provided on the following page.

Chapter Three: How to Prepare Tea

<u>To make your own tea bags, simply follow the steps outlined below:</u>

Materials Required:

- 1 cup dried loose leaf tea
- Cone-style coffee filters
- Thin cotton string
- Stapler or needle and thread

Instructions:

1. Choose a loose leaf tea that you enjoy and make sure that it is properly dried and ready to use.
2. If you like, you can combine several different types of loose leaf tea to make your own individual flavour profiles.
3. Cut each of your coffee filters in half from top to bottom then trim about 1 inch off the top of each half.
4. Spoon about 1 teaspoon of your loose leaf tea into each half cone then fold the open side over itself several times to close it.
5. Fold the top corners of the packet in toward the centre then fold the top down over them.

Chapter Three: How to Prepare Tea

6. Cut your string into 4-inch lengths and place the end of one string in the middle of the folded-down top of each tea bag.
7. Staple the end of the string in place or sew it down using a needle and thread.
8. If you like, you can create paper labels for your tea bags and staple them to the other end of the string.
9. Store your tea bags in an airtight container and use them as you would a normal tea bag.

Not only are these homemade tea bags a great way to make your own individual tea combinations, but they make excellent gifts as well!

Chapter Four: Health Benefits of Tea

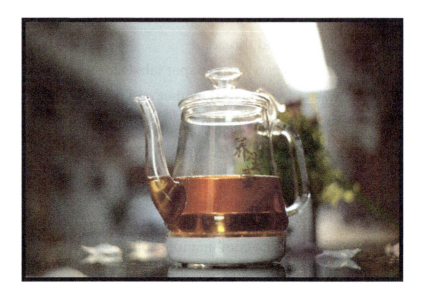

As you already know, tea is one of the most popular beverages in the world, and for good reason. Tea provides a wide variety of health benefits. People who drink tea regularly, for example, may have a lower risk for cardiovascular disease and diabetes. Tea is loaded with a number of health-promoting substances including catechins, polyphenols, epicatechins, antioxidants, and more. As an added bonus, it is extremely low in calories with just a few calories per cup (unsweetened).

Chapter Four: Health Benefits of Tea

1.) Top 10 Health Benefits of Tea

Drinking tea provides a wide variety of health benefits. <u>Below you will find a list of the top ten benefits associated with drinking tea</u>:

1. The antioxidants in green tea can help boost your exercise endurance – they also help your body to burn fat as fuel which helps with improved muscle endurance.

2. Tea has a high oxygen redial absorbance capacity (ORAC) which means that it helps to destroy free radicals in the body. Free radicals can damage your cells, causing serious health problems like heart disease, diabetes, and cancer.

3. Tea may help to protect you from damage caused by ultra-violet rays.

4. The antioxidants in tea may help to protect you against several types of cancer including colon, breast, skin, liver, pancreas, prostate, and oral cancers.

Chapter Four: Health Benefits of Tea

5. Drinking tea regularly may help to promote a healthy BMI and lower waist circumference – it also reduces your risk for metabolic syndrome.

6. Drinking tea regularly could counteract some of the negative side effects of smoking and could reduce your risk for lung cancer.

7. Those who drink tea regularly have a lower risk for neurodegenerative diseases like Parkinson's disease and Alzheimer's disease.

8. Individuals with diabetes may benefit from drinking tea regularly – it may help the body to process sugars more effectively.

9. Drinking tea can help the body to recover from radiation – it also helps to protect your cells against degeneration when exposed to radiation.

10. Certain types of tea (like green tea) have been shown to help improve both bone mineral density and strength.

Chapter Four: Health Benefits of Tea

2.) Tea Benefits for Weight Loss

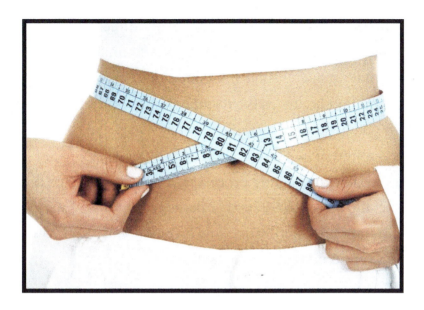

Tea is rich in polyphenols, an organic compound, which can help to increase your body's energy expenditure. When combined with the caffeine content of tea, these polyphenols help your body to burn more fat which can help you to lose weight or to maintain a healthy weight. In a research study conducted on green tea drinkers, subjects lost an average of 2.9 pounds over the course of 12 weeks while maintaining their normal diet. Other studies have shown that regular tea drinkers tend to have lower waist-to-hip ratios and lower body mass indexes (BMI).

Chapter Four: Health Benefits of Tea

3.) Tea Benefits for Inflammation

A wide variety of medical conditions are directly related to inflammation. There are two types of inflammation – acute inflammation and chronic inflammation. Acute inflammation occurs as the result of injury or trauma – when you get a cut or scrape, the area swells and turns red. This is a sign of increased blood flow to the area which helps to start the healing process and which also helps to protect the area against further damage. Chronic inflammation is long-lasting low level inflammation which can be very damaging to the body.

Chronic inflammation is linked to a number of serious health problems including the following:

- Asthma
- Tuberculosis
- Rheumatoid arthritis
- Chronic peptic ulcer
- Chronic sinusitis
- Ulcerative colitis
- Crohn's disease
- Chronic active hepatitis

This type of inflammation is also closely linked to autoimmune conditions like coeliac disease, type 1 diabetes, Addison's disease, and more.

Chapter Four: Health Benefits of Tea

Tea is rich in anti-inflammatory compounds and numerous studies have shown a link between drinking tea regularly and having a lower risk for inflammatory diseases. In these studies, regular drinkers of tea were found to have lower levels of nuclear factor kappa B (NFKB). This substance is a key indicator of the type of inflammation that has been linked to viral infections, autoimmune diseases, decreased immune development, and certain types of cancer. Studies have also shown that the polyphenol epigallocatechin-3-gallate (EGCG) reduces another type of protein, interleukin-8, which also causes inflammation.

Chapter Four: Health Benefits of Tea

4.) Tea Benefits for Mental Health

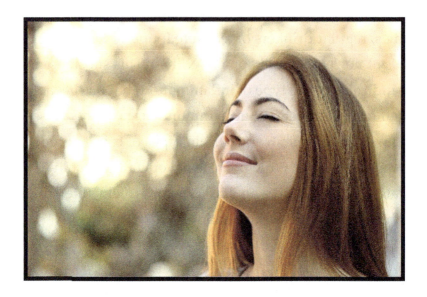

Drinking tea regularly can provide a number of benefits for your mental health. The polyphenol epigallocatechin-3-gallate (EGCG) has been shown to reduce the build-up of plaques in the brain which cause the cell death responsible for neurodegenerative diseases like Alzheimer's and Parkinson's disease. Tea also contains a psychoactive amino acid called theanine which increases cognitive performance. In a research study in which subjects drank two or three cups of tea within 90 minutes, those subjects were shown to be more alert and attentive to the study task than those who received a placebo drink.

Chapter Four: Health Benefits of Tea

Not only can drinking tea improve your cognitive performance, but it can also affect your mood and mental health. The same amino acid that leads to improved mental performance, theanine, has also been shown to provide a calming effect which is beneficial for individuals with anxiety and various mood disorders including schizophrenia. Theanine, along with EGCG, can also help to boost your memory by increasing your production of new brain cells.

Chapter Four: Health Benefits of Tea

5.) *Tea Benefits for Diabetes*

Tea contains a number of compounds which have been shown to have important health benefits for individuals with diabetes. Certain types of tea like green tea, black tea, and oolong tea contain polyphenols which have been shown to increase insulin activity in the body. Polyphenols have natural anti-oxidative properties as well, which can help to protect the body against inflammation. In a 2009 study, individuals who drank three cups of tea daily reduced their risk for type 2 diabetes by 40%.

Another way in which tea helps to prevent diabetes is by reducing an individual's risk for obesity – obesity is one of the most significant risk factors for diabetes. A 2013 research review that was published in the *Diabetes and Metabolism Journal* showed that individuals who drank 6 or more cups of green tea per day had a 33% reduced risk for developing type 2 diabetes. A Taiwanese study conducted over the course of a decade showed that tea drinkers had lower body fat percentages and smaller waists than those who did not drink tea.

Chapter Four: Health Benefits of Tea

6.) Tea Benefits for Heart Health

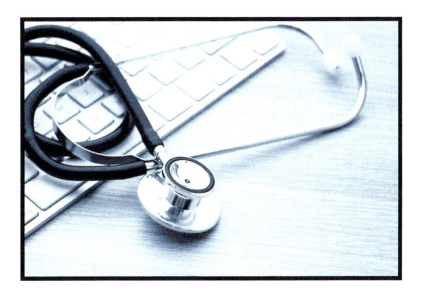

In addition to promoting mental health and a decreased risk for diabetes, polyphenols can also help to reduce oxidative stress. Oxidative stress can lead to vasodilation, or widening of the arteries, which leads to decreased blood pressure, reduced cholesterol, and problems with blood clotting. These three activities contribute to a reduced risk for cardiovascular disease.

According to a 2012 study published in Food & Function, drinking black or green tea can help reduce the risk of coronary heart disease and stroke by as much as 20%. In 2010, a large study published in Arteriosclerosis, Thrombosis and Vascular Biology followed 37,000 study participants over the course of 13 years. Study participants who drank between 3 and 6 cups of tea daily had a 45% reduced risk of dying from heart disease. Several studies have also linked the anti-inflammatory benefits provided by the antioxidant EGCG to reduced risk for atherosclerosis, largely because it helps to reduce plaque build-up in both the bloodstream and in arterial walls.

Chapter Four: Health Benefits of Tea

7.) Tea Health Benefits Chart

Different kinds of tea provide different health benefits. Below you will find a chart detailing the four types of tea made from the *Camellia sinensis* plant which provide certain health benefits:

Benefit	Green	Black	White	Oolong
Anti-Aging	X		X	X
Improved Cognitive Focus/Alertness	X	X		X
Improved Digestive Health		X		
Improved Glucose Metabolism	X			
Improved Immune System Health	X	X	X	
Increased Fat Burning	X			X
Kills Free Radicals	X			X
Lowers Blood Cholesterol	X			
Reduces Risk for Heart Disease	X	X	X	
Reduces Risk for Osteoporosis	X	X		X
Reduces Risk for Stroke		X		
Relief from Skin Problems				X
Relieves Anxiety and Stress		X		X

Chapter Four: Health Benefits of Tea

Relieves Arthritis Pain	X			
Rich in Antioxidants	X	X	X	
Prevents Neurodegenerative Disease	X			
Prevents Skin Damage	X		X	X
Promotes Weight Loss	X		X	X
Protects Oral Health		X	X	X
Stabilizes Blood Lipid Levels	X			
Suppresses Cancer Growth	X	X		X

Chapter Five: Types of Tea

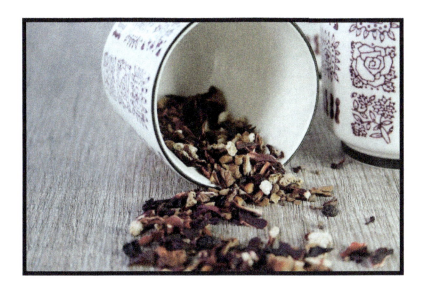

If you walk into a tea shop you might easily be overwhelmed by the sheer number of options available to you. Tea comes in many different flavours, each with its own unique aroma and taste. Technically there are only four types of "real" tea – those derived from the *Camellia sinensis* plant. These varieties include green, black, white, and oolong tea. Teas made from other plants, like herbal teas, are technically infusions, not tea. In this chapter you will receive an overview of some of the most popular types of tea available.

Chapter Five: Types of Tea

a.) Green Tea

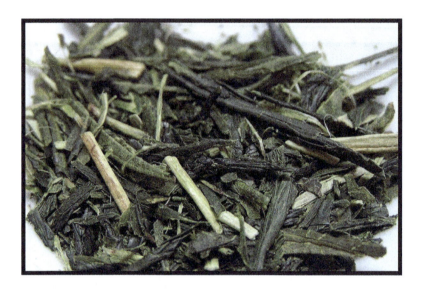

Plant Used: *Camellia sinensis*

Country of Origin: China

Category: Green

Water Temperature: 160° to 180°F (71° to 82°C)

Infusion Time: 2 to 3 minutes

Green tea is the most popular form of tea consumed in China and it has been associated with many other Asian cultures as well. This type of tea can be brewed using about 2 grams of tea per 100ml of water (about one teaspoon per

Chapter Five: Types of Tea

5-ounce cup). There are more than 600 different cultivars of the *Camellia sinensis* plant which can be used to make different varieties of green tea.

The consumption of green tea has been linked to many significant health benefits. Not only can drinking green tea reduce your risk for cancer, heart disease, and stroke, but it also promotes healthy weight loss and weight maintenance. Green tea can also help diabetics to process sugar more effectively and it may help to decrease LDL cholesterol levels as well.

Varieties of Green Tea Include:

- Lonjing
- Jasmine Tea
- Sencha
- Matcha

Health Benefits of Green Tea Include:

- Contains antioxidants called catechins which kill free radicals and help to prevent wrinkling and skin damage.
- May suppress the growth of cancer cells and provide protection against carcinogens.

Chapter Five: Types of Tea

- Improves glucose and lipid metabolism to prevent sharp spikes in blood sugar levels.
- Promotes weight loss by increasing fat burning in the body, especially in the abdominal area.
- May help ease the pain of rheumatoid arthritis and fractures caused by osteoporosis.
- Enzymes in green tea reduce the risk for brain cell damage – may help prevent Alzheimer's and Parkinson's disease.
- Helps to ward off infection and allergies.
- May help lower/stabilize blood cholesterol levels in the body.

Chapter Five: Types of Tea

Jasmine Tea

This type of tea can be made with several kinds of tea, but it is most commonly made with black tea. Jasmine tea is simply black tea that has been scented with the aroma of jasmine blossoms. This kind of tea has a strong fragrance and a subtly sweet flavour – it is the most famous scented tea found in China. The health benefits of jasmine tea depend on the type of tea used to make it, but the jasmine scent itself may providing relaxing effects.

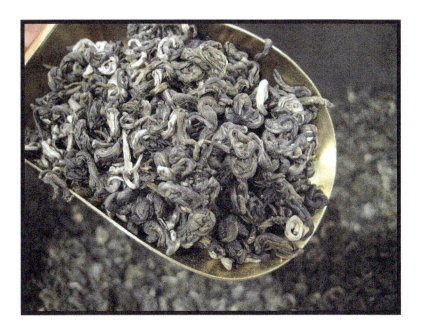

Figure 1: Jasmine Tea

Chapter Five: Types of Tea

Lonjing

This type of tea has been pan-roasted and it is sometimes referred to as Dragon Well tea. Longjing tea originated in the Longjing Village area in Zhejiang Province, China. This type of tea is widely known for its high quality and it is minimally oxidized. Longjing tea contains valuable amino acids as well as vitamin C – it also has one of the highest concentrations of catechins of any tea.

Matcha

This green tea variety goes through a special growth and processing method. The tea plants are grown in the shade for about 3 weeks before being harvested, and the stems and veins of the leaves are removed before they are processed. By growing the plants in the shade, matcha tea has higher concentrations of theanine and chlorophyll – both of these compounds help to improve mental focus. Matcha tea is stone-ground into a powder after drying and it can be prepared thick or thin, depending on the amount of water used to prepare it.

Chapter Five: Types of Tea

Sencha

This type of tea is prepared by boiling whole tea leaves in hot water and it is the most popular type of tea in Japan. Sencha tea varies in flavour depending where it is produced, but the first harvest of the season – called "shincha", or 'new tea – is considered to be the most flavourful and delicious. Sencha leaves are steamed before being dried unlike Chinese green teas which are pan-fired.

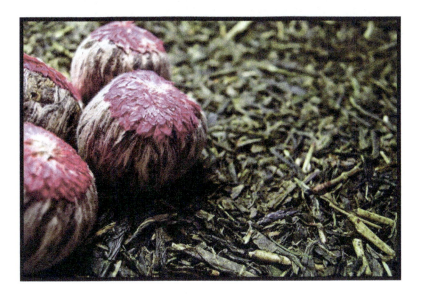

Figure 2: Sencha and Blooming Jasmine Tea

Chapter Five: Types of Tea

b.) Black Tea

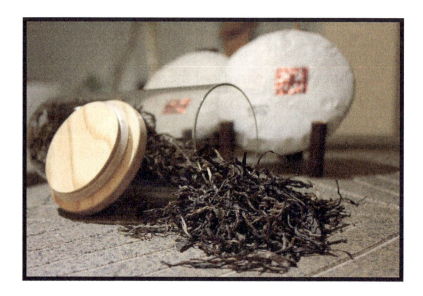

Plant Used: *Camellia sinensis* subsp. *sinensis*, subsp. *assamica*

Country of Origin: China

Category: Black

Water Temperature: 212°F (100°C)

Infusion Time: 4 to 6 minutes

Black tea is the most commonly consumed type of tea in the West and it comes in many different varieties. This type of tea is typically stronger in flavour than other teas and it has the ability to retain its flavour for several years. In China,

Japan, Korea, and other Asian countries, black tea is commonly known as "red" tea due to the colour of the liquid. In Western cultures, the term "black tea" refers to the dark colour of the leaves. In China, the term "black tea" refers to a classification for post-fermented teas like Pu-erh.

This type of tea is more highly oxidized than green, white, and oolong tea and it has a stronger flavour. Black tea accounts for more than 90% of tea sold in the West, though green tea has recently seen a revival in popularity. This type of tea differs in flavour depending on the region in which it is produced.

Varieties of Black Tea Include:

- Almond Tea
- Assam
- Darjeeling
- Ceylon
- Masala Tea

Black tea can also be mixed with different plants or substances to create different flavours including:

- **Earl Grey** – Black tea mixed with bergamot oil
- **Masala chai** – Blend of black tea, spices, milk, and sweetener

- **English Breakfast Tea** – Blended to go with milk and sugar; full-bodied and robust/rich
- **English Afternoon Tea** - Blended with Ceylon; medium-bodied and bright
- **Irish Breakfast Tea** – Blend of several black teas, typically Assam and others

Health Benefits of Black Tea Include:

- This type of tea may help to reduce plaque formation and to reduce bacteria growth which may cause cavities.
- Consumption of black tea has been linked to reduced risk for stroke.
- This type of tea is rich in polyphenols, a type of antioxidant which helps to block the DNA damage caused by smoking and other chemicals.
- Black tea may help to reduce cancer growth and could help prevent certain types of cancer including ovarian cancer.
- Drinkers or black tea tend to have stronger bones and a reduced risk for arthritis and osteoporosis.
- Black tea provides stress-relieving benefits – the theanine content not only helps you relax, but it boosts your mental concentration as well.
- Alkylamine antigens in black tea help to boost your immune response for improved protection against common viruses.

Chapter Five: Types of Tea

- The tannins found in black tea may help to improve digestive health and to reduce digestive illnesses.
- Though much lower in caffeine than coffee, black tea helps to increase blood flow to the brain for boosted energy without over-stimulating your heart.

Chapter Five: Types of Tea

Assam

This type of tea is named after the region in which it is produced – Assam, India. Assam tea is produced from a cultivar of the tea plant, *Camellia sinensis* var. *assamica*. This kind of tea is known for its malty flavour and strong colour. The malty flavour is due to the tropical climate in which this type of tea is grown. Assam teas are typically sold as "breakfast" teas like Irish breakfast tea.

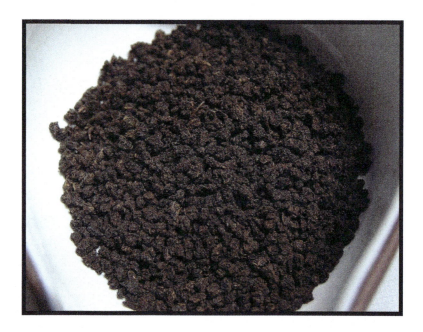

Figure 3: Assam Tea

Chapter Five: Types of Tea

Almond Tea

This type of tea can be made from a variety of teas, but black tea is the most common. Almond tea is simply tea that has been flavoured with almond. Almond tea has a pleasant almond aroma with a nutty, slightly sweet flavour. The almond flavour may help to balance out the astringency of black tea.

Darjeeling

This black tea variety comes from the Darjeeling district in West Bengal, India. Darjeeling tea is made from a different tea cultivar than most Indian teas – it is made from the Chinese tea plant, *Camellia sinensis* var. *sinensis*. This type of tea was first produced in 1841 and it is now available in several varieties including white, green, and oolong. Many Darjeeling teas are actually a blend of black, green, and oolong teas based on the level of oxidation.

Ceylon

This type of tea is named for the area in which it was first produced – Ceylon, now known as Sri Lanka. Ceylon tea is a high-quality tea with a crisp citrus-like aroma. This type of tea is used alone and in blends – it also comes in green and white varieties.

Chapter Five: Types of Tea

Masala Tea

Also known as masala chai, this type of tea is actually a blended tea beverage consisting of brewed black tea mixed with Indian herbs and spices. It is also often mixed with milk or cream. Masala tea originated in India but it is popular around the world, featured in many tea houses and coffee shops. This type of tea is traditionally prepared with a decoction of herbs including cinnamon sticks, ground cloves, ginger, black peppercorn, and cardamom pods. Today, however, it is available in tea bags and powdered mixes or concentrates.

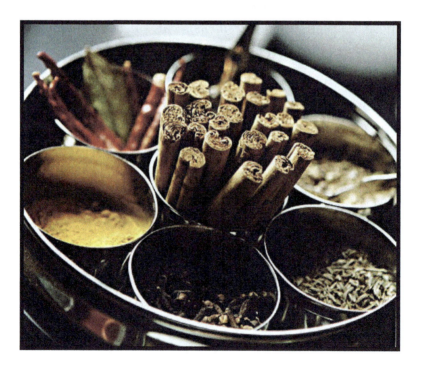

c.) White Tea

Plant Used: *Camellia sinensis*

Country of Origin: China

Category: White

Water Temperature: 150° to 160°F (65° to 71°C)

Infusion Time: 2 minutes

The name "white tea" is given in references to the silver-white hairs found on the unopened bud of the Camellia sinensis plant – these hairs give the plant a whitish colour. When brewed, white tea is not actually white or colourless, it is more of a pale yellow. White tea is grown and harvested primarily in China, specifically within the Fujian province.

There is a great deal of debate regarding the first production of white tea, though it is commonly believed to have been created within the last two centuries. It may have been first mentioned in an English publication from 1876 where it was classified as a black tea because it wasn't cooked initially like green tea. This type of tea shares many of the same benefits as green and black tea because it is made from the same plant – it has a higher antioxidant content than either of the other two, however.

Health Benefits of White Tea Include:

- This type of tea contains the same kinds of antioxidants as green tea, but in much higher concentrations.
- The caffeine content of white tea is less than coffee but it has been shown to help support healthy weight loss.
- The antioxidants found in white tea provide a number of anti-aging benefits by reducing free radical damage.
- White tea helps to support healthy, youthful-looking skin – it also protects skin from UV light.
- This type of tea provides oral health benefits by inhibiting the growth of cavity-causing bacteria and reducing plaque build-up.
- The flavonoids found in white tea may help decrease blood pressure which helps reduce your risk for cardiovascular disease.
- White tea has natural antibacterial properties which can help protect you against infection.

Chapter Five: Types of Tea

d.) Oolong Tea

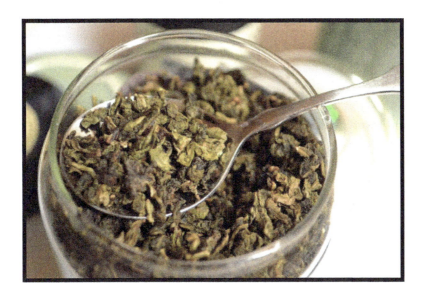

Plant Used: *Camellia sinensis*

Country of Origin: China

Category: Oolong

Water Temperature: 190° to 203°F (88° to 95°C)

Infusion Time: 3 to 4 minutes

Oolong tea is a type of traditional Chinese tea that is produced by withering the *Camellia sinensis* plant under the sun before the leaves are curled and twisted. The degree of oxidation for oolong tea ranges from as low as 8% to as high as 85% and unique cultivars of the *Camellia sinensis* plant are used to create specific Oolong varieties. The taste of oolong tea varies according to the cultivar used.

Many oolong teas have a sweet and fruity aroma, though some have a woody or earthy smell. Different cultivars are processed differently but there are only two methods of leaf formation. Some leaves are rolled into long curls and others are wrapped into small beads with tails. The first style is more commonly used in China.

Health Benefits of Oolong Tea Include:

- The polyphenols found in oolong tea may help to increase fat burning and it supports healthy body weight.
- Antioxidants found on oolong tea (primarily polyphenols) also help to remove free radicals which are responsible for skin damage, cancer, arthritis, and more.
- Drinking oolong tea may help to provide relief from skin-related health problems including eczema.
- The antioxidants in oolong tea not only help protect your teeth from decay, but they may help strengthen your bones to prevent osteoporosis

Chapter Five: Types of Tea

- Drinking oolong tea may help to reduce your risk for certain types of cancers – it may also inhibit the growth of cancer cells.
- Oolong tea contains an amino acid called L-theanine which helps to reduce stress levels.
- Drinking oolong tea may boost your concentration and mental performance/alertness.

Chapter Five: Types of Tea

e.) Herbal Tea

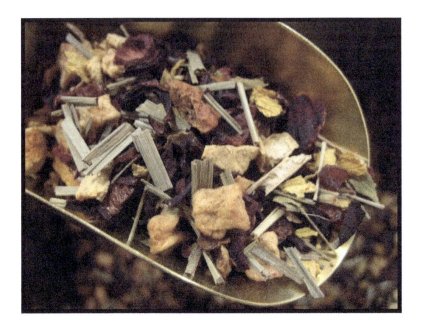

Plant Used: Varied

Country of Origin: China

Category: Herbal

Water Temperature: boiling

Infusion Time: 4 to 6 minutes

The name "herbal tea" is given to any beverage made from the decoction or infusion of spices, herbs, or other plant materials in hot water. Technically, it is not a type of tea because it is not made from the *Camellia sinensis* plant. Another distinguishing feature of herbal teas is that they typically do not contain caffeine. In some cultures, the word "tea" is only used in reference to the leaves of the *Camellia sinensis* plant so the term "herbal tea" is not used. Rather, this kind of beverage is called an infusion or a tisane.

Herbal teas have been in existence for as long as written history can account for. These teas can be served hot or cold and they provide a wide variety of health benefits depending on the plant from which they are brewed. The flavour and aroma of herbal teas varies according to the plant used as well.

Chapter Five: Types of Tea

Varieties of Herbal Tea Include:

- Barley Tea
- Calendula Tea
- Chaga Tea
- Chamomile/Camomile Tea
- Catnip Tea
- Cinnamon Tea
- Coca Tea
- Comfrey Tea
- Corn Silk Tea
- Damiana Tea
- Dandelion Tea
- Echinacea Tea
- Fennel Tea
- Fenugreek Tea
- Ginger Tea
- Gingko Biloba Tea
- Ginseng Tea
- Graviola Tea
- Hibiscus Tea
- Holy Basil Tea
- Honeybush Tea
- Horsetail Tea
- Kava Tea
- Lemon Balm Tea
- Licorice/Liquorice
- Mint Tea
- Moringa Tea
- Mother's Milk Tea
- Mulberry Tea
- Mullein Tea
- Nettle Tea
- Parsley Tea
- Poppy Seed Tea
- Raspberry Tea
- Red Bush Tea
- Red Clover Tea
- Rooibos Tea
- Rosehip Tea
- Saffron Tea
- Sage Tea
- Sassafras Tea
- Senna Tea
- Tulsi Tea
- Turmeric Tea
- Yarrow Tea

Chapter Five: Types of Tea

Barley Tea

Also known as roasted barley tea, this type of tea is an infusion made from the barley grain. This type of tea is particularly popular in Chinese, Korean, and Japanese cultures – it has also been used as a coffee substitute in the United States. Barley tea is called "mugicha" in Japanese, "maicha" in Chinese, and "boricha" in Korean. This type of tea may provide oral health benefits by helping to prevent tooth decay and bacterial growth – it may also help to reduce the risk for cardiovascular disease.

Catnip Tea

This type of tea is brewed from the flowers and leaves of the catnip (*Nepeta cataria*) plant, also known as catmint. Catnip tea contains nepetalactone which causes euphoria in house cats – in humans, it has a mildly sedative effect. In some cases, catnip tea may also be effective in treating or preventing inflammation.

Calendula Tea

This type of tea is made from an infusion of the flowers of the calendula plant (*Calendula officinalis*). Calendula tea is commonly used to treat muscle spasms and menstrual cramps but it can also help to reduce fever, to soothe sore throat, and to reduce inflammatory skin conditions. This tea

Chapter Five: Types of Tea

can also be applied topically as an herbal remedy for skin problems, flea bites, and minor wounds.

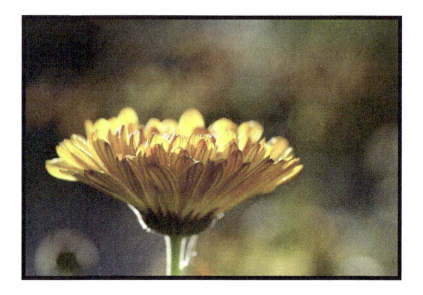

Figure 4: Calendula

Chaga Tea

This type of tea is brewed from the chaga mushroom (*Inonotus obliquus*), which is a type of fungus commonly found growing on birch treas. Chaga tea is a common Russian folk remedy that has been used since the 16th century for its antioxidant and anti-inflammatory benefits. This type of tea may also help to prevent cardiovascular disease, diabetes, and cancer. Because the chaga mushroom many interact with certain drugs, always check with your physician before drinking it.

Chamomile /Camomile Tea
This type of tea is brewed from the dried flowers of the German chamomile (*Matricaria chamomilla*) plant. This herbal tea is commonly used to promote sleep, though it can also help relieve stomach upset and constipation. Chamomile tea should be steeped for 10 to 15 minutes which is longer than most herbal teas, and it should remain covered to avoid dissipation of the volatile oils.

Cinnamon Tea
This type of tea is brewed from the bark of the cinnamon tree (*Cinnamomum verum*). Cinnamon tea has natural anti-viral, anti-fungal, and anti-bacterial properties so it may help to boost your immune system. This type of tea also helps to relieve symptoms of inflammatory conditions including arthritis. Cinnamon tea is rich in antioxidants which may help to prevent chronic medical problems like cardiovascular disease, diabetes, and stroke.

Chapter Five: Types of Tea

Coca Tea

This herbal tea is made by infusing the leaves of the coca plant (*Erythroxylum coca*) which is native to South America. Coca tea has a mildly bitter flavour which is similar to green tea and it has a greenish yellow colour. This type of tea contains alkaloids in low levels which act as a mild stimulant. The most common use for this tea is as an altitude sickness preventive. Because coca tea is made from the same plant as the drug cocaine, drinking non-decocainised coca tea may result in a positive drug test result with just one cup.

Comfrey Tea

This type of tea is made from the dried leaves of the comfrey plant (*Symphytum officinale*). This herbal tea has been used to promote the healing of broken bones, sprains, and arthritis. It may also stimulate cell repair and growth while also reducing inflammation. The safety of comfrey tea consumption is widely debated – some scientists maintain that it is only safe for topical use.

Corn Silk Tea

This type of tea is made from fresh or dried corn silk and it is a natural herbal remedy used by Native Americans. Corn silk tea has natural antiseptic properties which can help with kidney and bladder problems as well as urinary tract infections. This type of tea may help to flush out retained water and it may help children stop wetting the bed.

Damiana Tea
This tea is made from the leaves and flowers of the damiana shrub (*Turnera diffusa*). This type of tea has natural relaxation benefits similar to chamomile and it has long been claimed to have an aphrodisiac effect. Damiana tea may also help to reduce anxiety and menstrual cramps.

Echinacea Tea
This herbal tea is brewed from the flowers of the Echinacea plant (*Echinacea purpurea*). This tea is commonly reported to be beneficial in treating the common cold, though scientific evidence supporting this claim is weak. In general, Echinacea tea is said to help boost the immune system in fighting common infections.

Dandelion Tea
Also known as dandelion coffee, dandelion tea is brewed from the root of the dandelion (*Taraxacum officinale*) plant.

This type of tea has a bitter flavour similar in appearance and taste to coffee. Dandelion tea is reported to be a good tonic for the liver and it may be used as a natural laxative. Current research is underway regarding the potential benefits of dandelion tea for cancer treatment.

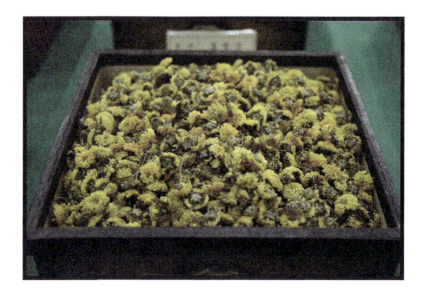

Figure 5: Dandelion Tea

Fennel Tea

This type of tea is brewed from the seeds of the fennel plant (*Foeniculum vulgare*), a flowering perennial herb. Fennel tea is highly flavourful and aromatic, similar in taste to anise tea. This herbal tea helps to reduce bloating and flatulence and it may also help to reduce symptoms related to irritable bowel syndrome (IBS). Fennel tea may help to relieve sore throat, lower blood pressure, and reduce pain caused by inflammatory conditions like rheumatoid arthritis.

Fenugreek Tea

This type of tea is made from the seeds of the fenugreek plant (*Trigonella foenum-graecum*), an annual herb. This herb was commonly used in ancient Egypt and it continues to play a large role in Mediterranean cuisine. Fenugreek tea may help to increase the milk supply of breastfeeding women and it helps to encourage healthy blood flow and circulation. This type of tea may be used as a digestive aid to relieve constipation, stomach ache, and nausea.

Ginger Tea

This herbal tea is made from the rhizome of the ginger root plant (*Zingiber officinale*) which is a flowering plant native to China. Ginger has a hot flavour and a strong aroma and, when served in tea, it is often sweetened with honey. Ginger tea provides a number of health benefits such as fighting cancer, reducing symptoms of IBS, and protecting your brain against neurodegenerative disease. Regularly drinking ginger tea may also help to promote weight loss and to increase nutrient absorption.

Gingko Biloba Tea

This type of tea is made from the gingko biloba tree (*Gingko biloba*) which is native to China and is said to be the oldest tree on earth. Gingko biloba tea contains high levels of antioxidants which may help to prevent cancer, reduce free radical damage, and to slow the signs of aging. This herbal tea may also help to stimulate blood circulation and reduce plaque build-up in the arteries to help prevent cardiovascular disease.

Ginseng Tea

This herbal tea is made from the root of the ginseng plant (*Panax ginseng*) which is found throughout North America and in parts of eastern Asia. Ginseng tea has been used in folk medicine as a stimulant and an aphrodisiac – it is also a common ingredient in energy drinks. Other uses for ginseng tea include boosting the immune system, relieving sexual disorders, aiding digestion, and reducing pain related to arthritis.

Chapter Five: Types of Tea

Graviola Tea

This tea is made from the leaf of the graviola tree (*Annona muricata*), also known as the soursop tree. This herbal tea has been shown to have powerful anti-cancer properties and it has been used to treat viral infections. Graviola tea may help to reduce pain and swelling as well.

Holy Basil Tea

(See Tulsi Tea)

Honeybush Tea

The leaves of the honeybush plant (*Cyclopia intermedia*), a plant belonging to the legume family, are used to produce honeybush tea. This herbal tea is similar to rooibos tea and it is only produced in a few small areas in South Africa. Honeybush tea is a little sweeter than rooibos tea and, unlike traditional teas, it doesn't turn sour with prolonged steeping or simmering. This tea has calming effects which are beneficial for individuals suffering from anxiety and insomnia. It also contains a variety of antioxidants.

Hibiscus Tea

This herbal tea is made from the flowers of the hibiscus plant (*Hibiscus syriacus*). Hibiscus tea is served around the world in both hot and cold forms, known not only for its colour but its rich, tangy flavour. This herbal tea is a natural diuretic which can help flush retained water from the body. It may also help reduce blood pressure which could reduce your risk for heart disease.

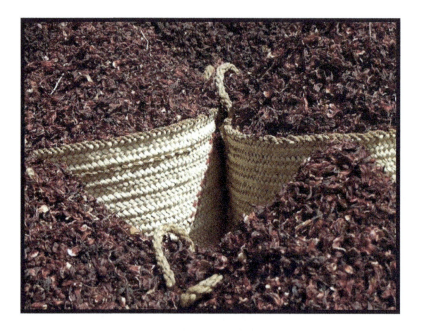

Figure 6: Hibiscus Tea

Horsetail Tea

This type of tea is made from the horsetail plant (genus *Equisetum*) which are one of the oldest living groups of plants. Horsetail tea was used by the ancient Greeks and

Romans to stop bleeding, to heal ulcers, and to treat kidney conditions. Today, horsetail tea is reported to help improve bone, skin and hair health – it may also be beneficial for healthy weight control.

Kava Tea

This herbal tea is made from the roots of the kava plant (*Piper methysticum*) which is native to the western Pacific region. Kava tea is known for its anaesthetic and sedative properties so it is a common treatment for anxiety and insomnia. The active compounds in kava tea are called kavalactones and they affect the levels of neurotransmitters in the blood.

Lemon Balm Tea

This herbal tea is made from the lemon balm plant (*Melissa officinalis*), a perennial herb belonging to the mint family. This tea has a calming effect which is beneficial for individuals suffering from anxiety or insomnia. It may also help to stimulate digestion and ease gastrointestinal issues. When applied topically, lemon balm tea helps to relieve skin problems.

Liquorice/Licorice Tea

This herbal tea is made from the root of the liquorice plant (*Glycyrrhia glabra*) which is technically a type of legume. Liquorice tea has a strong flavour similar to anise and fennel tea due to the presence of anethole and glycyrrhizin compounds. This type of tea has expectorant properties and can thus be used to soothe respiratory conditions like sore throat, coughing, bronchitis, and congestion. Liquorice tea may also help to treat digestive issues.

Mint Tea

Herbal tea can be made from several varieties of mint including spearmint and peppermint. Mint tea provides a variety of benefits such as improving digestion, reducing inflammation, relaxing the mind and body, and boosting the immune system. Mint tea may also have a cooling effect which can be used to relieve fever.

Moringa Tea

This type of tea is made from the dried leaves of the moringa plant (*Moringa oleifera*), a flowering plant native to parts of Asia and Africa. The leaves of this plant are often fed to cattle to increase weight and milk production. For humans, moringa tea can help to boost the immune system, support brain and eye health, increase metabolism, and promote healthy liver and kidney function. Moringa tea also provides anti-inflammatory benefits.

Mother's Milk Tea

(See Fenugreek Tea)

This type of tea is made with fenugreek as the main ingredient and its main benefit is to help increase milk supply in breastfeeding women.

Mulberry Tea

This type of herbal tea is made from the fruit of the mulberry tree (*Morus alba*). Mulberry tea can be used to relieve cold symptoms and to reduce high blood pressure. It is also said to naturally inhibit carbohydrate absorption which may result in weight loss. Mulberry tea helps to maintain balanced blood sugar levels and it reduces the risk for atherosclerosis by maintaining blood vessel health.

Mullein Tea

This tea is made from the leaves of the mullein plant (*Verbascum thapsus*), a flowering plant native to parts of Asia and Europe. This herbal tea is commonly used as a mucilage to relieve respiratory conditions like bronchitis, congestion, and asthma. Mullein tea may also help to relieve diarrhoea and intestinal inflammation.

Nettle Tea

This type of tea is made from the nettle, or stinging nettle, plant (*Urtica dioica*). Nettle tea was historically used as an herbal remedy or folk remedy for a variety of conditions including arthritis, digestive disorders, headache, and respiratory conditions. Today, nettle tea is commonly used for its anti-inflammatory, diuretic, and astringent benefits.

Parsley Tea

This type of tea is made from the parsley herb (*Petroselinum crispum*) which is native to the Mediterranean region but cultivated throughout the world. Parsley tea has been used as an herbal remedy for centuries due to its strong immune-boosting benefits. This herbal tea contains flavonoids as well as powerful antioxidants which can help prevent free radical damage to your cells. Regular consumption of parsley tea may help to regulate menstrual periods and to promote uterine contractions following childbirth. Parsley tea can be helpful in treating kidney conditions and for reducing water retention.

Chapter Five: Types of Tea

Poppy Seed Tea

Also known simply as poppy tea, poppy seed tea is made from the straw or seeds of the poppy plant (*Papaver somniferum*). Poppy tea contains opiate alkaloids including morphine which produce a narcotic effect. This herbal tea can be consumed in small amounts for its anti-diarrheal, sedative, and analgesic effects.

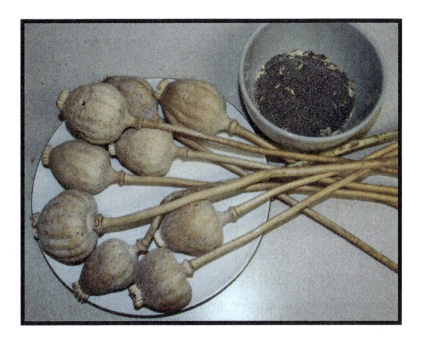

Figure 7: Poppy Seed Tea

Raspberry Tea

Also known as red raspberry leaf tea, raspberry tea is made from the leaf produced by the raspberry plant (*Rubus idaeus*). This tea is rich in tannins as well as various vitamins and minerals. The most common use for raspberry leaf tea is to ease the symptoms of premenstrual syndrome. Historically, raspberry leaf tea was used to aid childbirth delivery and treat cold sores, leg cramps, diarrhoea, morning sickness, anaemia, and canker sores.

Red Bush Tea

(See Rooibos Tea)

Red Clover Tea

This herbal tea is made from the leaves and flowers of the red clover plant (*Trifolium pretense*) which is native to parts of Europe, Asia, and Africa. This herbal tea has a sweet flavour and it was used historically for its sedative, antispasmodic, expectorant, and anti-inflammatory benefits. This tea can be used to relieve respiratory conditions like bronchitis and asthma.

Rooibos Tea

The name rooibos translates to "red bush" and it refers to a member of the legume family native to South Africa called *Aspalathus linearis*. Rooibos tea has been called bush tea and redbush tea (particularly in Britain) and, though it is most common in South Africa, it is consumed around the world. This type of tea is consumed in a similar manner to black tea, often taken with sugar and milk. Rooibos tea can help to treat headache, insomnia, allergies, and skin conditions.

Rosehip Tea

Rosehip tea is made using the fruit of the rose plant (genus *Rosa*) and it contains high levels of various antioxidants including phenols and flavonoids. This herbal tea has been used to treat inflammatory conditions like rheumatoid arthritis and osteoporosis. Rosehips are often blended with hibiscus to make tea.

Saffron Tea

This herbal tea is made from the flower of the saffron plant (*Crocus sativus*). Saffron tea was historically treasured by the ancient Greeks, Romans and Egyptians, commonly used for culinary and medicinal purposes. Today, saffron tea helps to support eye health and it may offer anti-cancer benefits.

Saffron tea may also reduce your risk for cardiovascular disease thanks to its high concentration of the flavonoid lycopene (also found in tomatoes).

Sage Tea
This type of tea is made from the leaves of the sage plant (*Salvia officinalis*), a perennial herb native to the Mediterranean region. Sage tea contains polyphenols which may help to prevent cancer and it contains other antioxidants which support liver health. This herbal tea has been used to reduce anxiety and menopausal hot flashes.

Senna Tea
This type of tea is made from the senna plant (*Senna alexandrina*), a flowering plant found throughout the tropics. This type of tea has long been used in herbal remedies as a natural laxative. Overuse of this tea may result in diarrhoea and dehydration.

Chapter Five: Types of Tea

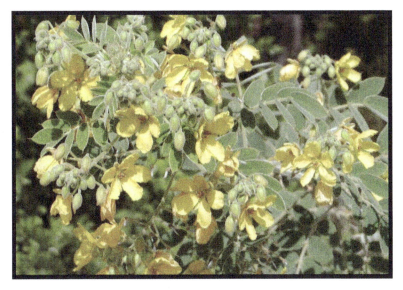

Figure 8: Senna

Sassafras Tea

This type of herbal tea is made from the bark of the sassafras tree (*Sassafras albidum*). Sassafras bark was widely used by the Native Americans to treat fever, urinary disorders, and skin conditions. Today, however, the volatile oils found in the root of the sassafras tree are known to contain a carcinogenic compound called safrole. Sassafras tea, however, is not dangerous though it is unlikely to provide any major health benefits.

Tulsi Tea

This type of tea is made from the leaves of the tulsi plant (*Ocimum tenuiflorum*) which is native to India. This plant is also known as "holy basil" and it is known for its essential oils. Tulsi tea may help to relieve the symptoms of respiratory conditions like cough and cold as well as asthma and bronchitis. This herbal tea is rich in magnesium which helps to prevent heart disease and it has natural stress-relieving properties. Tulsi tea also helps to inhibit bacterial growth which contribute to oral health problems.

Turmeric Tea

This herbal tea is made from the rhizomes of the turmeric plant (*Curcuma longa*) which is native to southwest India. Turmeric is known for its curcumin content provides antioxidant, antibacterial, antiviral, and anti-inflammatory benefits. Turmeric tea may help to prevent cardiovascular disease and certain types of cancer. This type of tea may also prevent the kind of neurodegeneration which is responsible for Alzheimer's disease.

Yarrow Tea

This herbal tea is made from the leaves of the yarrow plant (*Achillea millefolium*), a flowering plant native to the Northern Hemisphere. This tea can be used to reduce fever, to shorten the duration of colds, and to relieve cramps. It can even be applied topically to relieve itchy skin conditions. Yarrow tea has natural diuretic properties and it may support digestive health as well.

f.) Floral/Fruit Tea

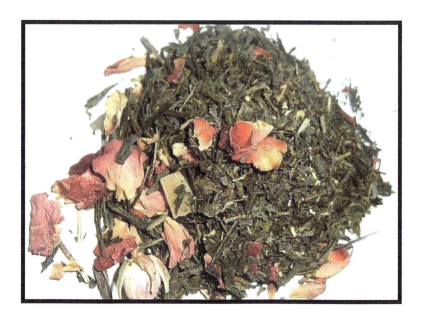

Plant Used: Varied

Category: Herbal

Water Temperature: boiling

Infusion Time: 4 to 6 minutes

Floral and fruit teas are simply a category of herbal teas. As you already know, herbal teas are infusions or decoctions made with plants other than the *Camellia sinensis* plant steeped in water. Floral teas like rose tea and linden tea are made using the petals of flowering plants while fruit teas are often brewed teas flavoured with specific fruits. Fruit teas can be made with nearly any variety of tea, though black tea is the most common. Many floral teas contain a variety of flavours and aromas all in one blend.

Varieties of Floral/Fruit Teas Include:

- Apple Tea
- Black Currant Tea
- Blueberry Tea
- Chrysanthemum Tea
- Cranberry Tea
- Lavender Tea
- Linden Tea
- Peach Tea
- Pineapple Tea
- Rose Tea
- Vanilla Tea

Chapter Five: Types of Tea

Apple Tea

This type of fruit tea can be made with several varieties of tea, but it is most commonly made with rooibos or black tea. Apple tea is available in tea bags or you can make your own by adding apple cider or apple juice to brewed tea. Apple tea is commonly flavoured with cinnamon.

Black Currant Tea

This type of tea is made from the fruit of the black currant plant (*Ribes nigrum*), a woody shrub native to northern Europe. Black currant tea is rich in vitamin C, a natural antioxidant which provides immune system benefits and protection against free radical damage. This type of tea can also be used for its anti-inflammatory and anti-viral benefits as well.

Blueberry Tea

The term "blueberry tea" technically refers to a cocktail made by adding brewed herbal tea to a combination of Grand Marnier and Amaretto liqueurs. Blueberry tea can also be a kind of herbal tea made with wild blueberries and blueberry leaves and other flavours.

Chapter Five: Types of Tea

Chrysanthemum Tea

This herbal tea is brewed from the chrysanthemum flower (*Chrysanthemum morifolium*). This type of tea is popular in East Asia and its use dates all the way back to the Song Dynasty (960 – 1279 AD). Chrysanthemum tea is a "cooling" herbal infusion which helps to relieve fever and sore throat – it can also be used to increase alertness. In ancient Chinese medicine, chrysanthemum tea was used to treat disorders of the liver and eyes.

Cranberry Tea

Like most fruit teas, cranberry tea can be made with several varieties of tea, but it is most commonly made with black tea. Cranberry tea is flavoured with dried cranberry which gives it a tangy flavour. This type of tea provides natural diuretic effects which can help your body to get rid of retained water.

Lavender Tea

This type of tea is a floral tea brewed using the dried flowers of the lavender herb (*Lavandula angustifolia*). Lavender comes from the mountains in the Mediterranean region but it is widely cultivated throughout the world. Lavender tea has a relaxing floral aroma that can be helpful for individuals suffering from stress, anxiety, depression, and insomnia. Lavender tea may also help relieve digestive issues like stomach upset and indigestion.

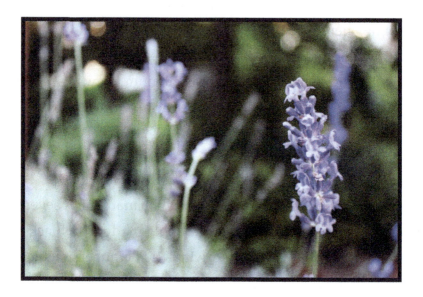

Figure 9: Lavender

Linden Tea

This type of tea is brewed from the dried flowers of the *Tilia platyphyllos* species, a flowering tree native to Europe. Linden tea has a mildly sweet taste and a floral aroma due to the volatile oils found in the linden flowers. This type of tea can be used to relieve cough, cold, fever, inflammation, and headache – it also acts as a natural diuretic and antispasmodic.

Peach Tea

Like apple and cranberry tea, peach tea can be made with several varieties of tea, but it is most commonly made with black tea. This type of herbal tea is flavoured with peach which not only gives it a fruity flavour, but a sweet and pleasing aroma as well.

Pineapple Tea

This kind of tea can be made with several types of tea, though black tea is most common. Pineapple tea consists of brewed tea blended with pineapple flavour from pureed pineapple, dried pineapple, or pineapple juice. Like cranberry tea, pineapple tea is a natural diuretic which can be used to relive water retention. Pineapple tea also has anti-inflammatory properties which can help to reduce swelling in cases of arthritis, sore throat, or gout.

Rose Tea

This kind of tea is brewed by steeping fresh or dried rose petals in hot water. Rose tea is a floral tea that has a floral aroma and a lightly sweet flavour. This type of tea provides a variety of benefits linked to its antioxidant content. Rose tea can be used to relieve menstrual cramps and it may help to boost your immune system due to its Vitamin C content. Rose tea is also rich in polyphenols which may help to reduce your risk for certain diseases like cancer and osteoporosis.

Vanilla Tea

This type of tea is commonly made with black tea and flavoured with dried or fresh vanilla beans. Vanilla tea typically has a rich, sweet aroma of vanilla – it may even smell like fresh-baked cookies. This kind of tea can be used to relieve nausea and it may help to support weight loss. Regular consumption of vanilla tea may also help to regulate the menstrual cycle for women.

Chapter Six: Where to Buy Tea

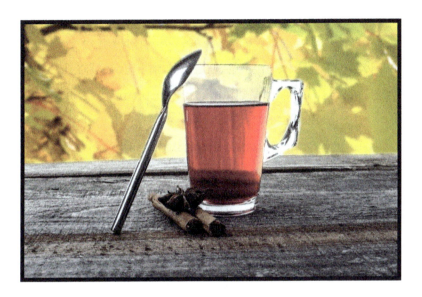

When it comes to buying tea, you have many options to choose from. You should be able to find a decent selection of tea bags at your local grocery store but, if you are looking for loose leaf tea or specialty teas, you may need to look elsewhere. One of the best places to buy tea is online because you can find large selections and low prices. In this chapter you will receive tips for purchasing tea online and for finding tea in your local area.

Chapter Six: Where to Buy Tea

1.) Tips for Buying Tea Online

If you cannot find a good selection of teas in your area, you may want to try buying tea online. The first thing you need to be aware of in buying tea online is that you should avoid the big chain stores – the chains that you find in shopping malls and tourist districts. These chains sell large quantities of low-quality tea purchased from brokers to keep their profit margins high. If you want to buy high-quality tea, look for a smaller supplier. These suppliers may not offer the same selection, but they are more likely to have higher quality tea.

When evaluating an online tea shop, take the time to read about the shop owner and his or her methods for collecting teas. Someone who flies around the world testing and buying teas will be a true believer in his or her product and you can bet that the tea is of high quality. There may only be a few varieties available each season, but they will be much better than anything you could buy from a chain store. You should also take the time to read the product descriptions on the site – look for descriptions of growing methods and processing methods to see if the company chooses its tea itself or if it is a generic product.

Chapter Six: Where to Buy Tea

Another thing to keep in mind when buying tea online is that tea is a seasonal product. Some teas age well but most teas should be enjoyed within a few months of being harvested. When evaluating a tea sale website, check to see if the stock rotates by season and look to see if the harvest dates are available. If you cannot find this information on the website, do not hesitate to call. If the website has a brick-and-mortar store, the employees will likely be happy to answer your questions.

One final thing to be ready for when shopping for tea online is the prices. High-quality tea can be expensive, though all expensive tea is not necessarily of high quality. Good quality tea leaves that are fresh from harvest and processed with care could cost as much as $500 (£325) or more per pound. Keep in mind, however, that you will only be using a small quantity of tea leaves per cup so your price per cup will only be about $0.50 (£0.32) if the tea costs $100 (£65) per pound.

Chapter Six: Where to Buy Tea

2. Recommended Online Suppliers

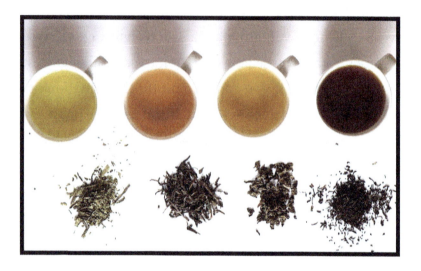

If you perform an online search for tea suppliers you will receive hundreds, even thousands of results. So how do you know if a supplier has high-quality tea? Reading the content on the website and calling to speak to someone at the company will help you to answer most of your questions.

If you are looking for some recommendations for good tea websites, consider some of the following:

Chapter Six: Where to Buy Tea

United States Suppliers

a.) Verdant Tea

The proprietor of this Minneapolis-based tea company, David Duckler, fell in love with Chinese tea culture while performing field research as an academic. This company maintains positive relationships with its farmers to provide fresh small-batch teas that hit the market just a few days after harvest. Stock is rotated every few weeks, not just once per season.

Website: http://verdanttea.com/

b. Crimson Lotus Tea

This Seattle-based company is run by husband and wife Glen Bowers and Dawa Lamu. This company is dedicated to selling unique pu-erhs, marketing their products specifically for new tea drinkers.

Website: http://crimsonlotustea.com/

c.) In Pursuit of Tea

This company is one of the few that offers a large selection of teas without sacrificing their quality. In Pursuit of Tea offers everything from Japanese teas to Himalayan teas as

Chapter Six: Where to Buy Tea

well as traditional Chinese options like pu-erhs and oolongs.

Website: http://www.inpursuitoftea.com/

d.) Red Blossom Tea Company

This San Francisco-based company offers a wide variety of Chinese teas, particularly some interesting flavours in both oolong and fermented teas.

Website: http://www.redblossomtea.com/

e.) Rishi

If you are looking for specialty blends or tea bags, Rishi has a very large selection. This is one of the few quality online suppliers that have made their way into several supermarkets – look for it at a store near you.

Website: http://www.rishi-tea.com/

Chapter Six: Where to Buy Tea

United Kingdom Suppliers

a.) Nothing But Tea

This website is run by a small group of tea professionals who dedicate their lives to the pursuit of good tea. Here you will find an assortment of loose leaf teas including black tea, green tea, and oolong teas as well as specialty teas like rooibos and herbal teas.

Website: http://nbtea.co.uk/store/

b.) Mad Hatter Tea

This company offers a unique assortment of Indian and African teas designed to offer both richness and a delicious depth of taste. Mad Hatter Tea is devoted to freshness and quality with each cup.

Website: http://www.madhattertea.co.uk/

c.) Jenier World of Teas

Based in Scotland, this company offers an extensive variety of teas available for delivery all over the world. This company has more than 30 years of experience producing and blending high-quality teas and they are devoted to

Chapter Six: Where to Buy Tea

providing quality products and excellent customer service. To get a 10% discount on your order just enter the code **TYPESOFTEA10** at the checkout.

Website: http://www.jenierteas.com/

d.) Tea Palace

A modern tea emporium located in London, England, the Tea Palace offers a wide selection of top-quality teas and infusions. This company is devoted to the rediscovery of the "proper cup of tea" by helping customers to not only find high-quality products but to educate them about where their teas come from and what benefits they provide.

Website: http://www.teapalace.co.uk/

e.) Drury Tea and Coffee Company

This family-owned business has a store in central London where they offer more than 100 varieties of tea. In addition to slow-roasting their own coffee blends, Drury employs a team of tea tasters to ensure the highest standards of quality for their products.

Website: http://www.drury.uk.com/

Chapter Six: Where to Buy Tea

3.) Finding a Local Tea Shop

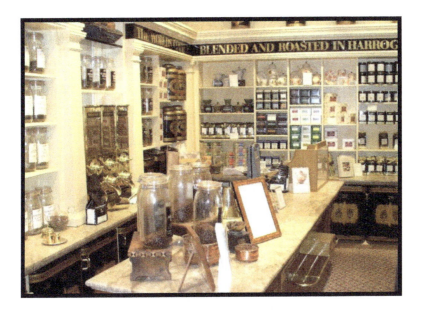

If you do not know what kind of tea you like, you may want to find a local tea house or tea shop where you can try a few different flavours before you buy. Ask around for recommendations or check the Yellow Pages or do an online search to find a tea shop near you. Small, locally-owned businesses are more likely to have high-quality loose leaf teas than chain stores. You will also be able to buy different teas in small quantities so you can try out as many flavours as you like.

Chapter Six: Where to Buy Tea

Another benefit to shopping at a local store is that the employees will be able to answer your questions. If you have some idea of what kind of tea you like, they will be able to help you find similar teas to try. You will also be able to find tea brewing equipment and accessories at a tea shop so, if you are looking for an infuser or a new teapot, this is a great place to look. You will also find many other tea enthusiasts with whom you can connect.

Conclusion

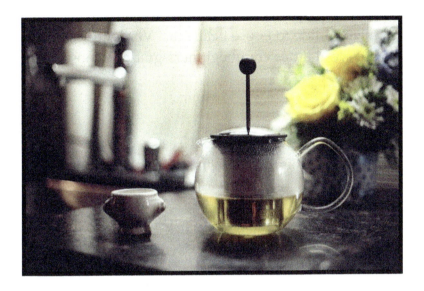

After reading this book you should have a deeper understanding – and hopefully a deeper appreciation – for tea. Not only is this beverage the most highly consumed beverage in the world (aside from water), but it is loaded with a variety of health benefits. Tea is packed with antioxidants and it has natural anti-inflammatory properties as well. Tea drinkers have also been found to have lower risk for diabetes and cardiovascular disease. If you aren't much of a tea drinker yet, you should consider giving it a try. There are many types to choose from so you can easily find one you like!

References

"Beginner's Guide to Loose Leaf Tea." Verdant Tea. <http://verdanttea.com/beginners-guide-to-loose-leaf-tea/#how>

"Brewing Methods." Mighty Leaf Tea. <http://www.mightyleaf.com/brewing-methods/>

Dhawan, Vibha. "11 Benefits of Black Tea that You Didn't Know About." LifeHack.org. < http://www.lifehack.org/articles/lifestyle/11-benefits-black-tea.html>

Edgar, Julie. "Types of Tea and Their Health Benefits." WebMD. <http://www.webmd.com/diet/tea-types-and-their-health-benefits>

Falkowitz, Max. "Where to Buy Amazing Tea Online." Serious Eats. <http://www.seriouseats.com/2015/02/best-tea-where-to-buy.html>

"Health Benefits of Tea." The Dr. Oz Show. <http://www.doctoroz.com/slideshow/health-benefits-tea?gallery=true&page=2>

"How to Make Tea Gongfu-Style." Verdant Tea. <http://verdanttea.com/tv/improvisational-gong-fu-tea/>

"How to Prepare the Perfect Cup of Green Tea." Itoen.co.jp. <http://www.itoen.co.jp/eng/allabout_greentea/how_to_prepare.html>

Lipoff, Sarah. "Homemade Tea Bags for Travel or Gifting." Popsugar. <http://www.popsugar.com/smart-living/DIY-Tea-Bags-32419246>

Newcomer, Laura. "13 Reasons Tea is Good for You." Time. <http://healthland.time.com/2012/09/04/13-reasons-to-love-tea/>

"Preparing Matcha Green Tea." TeaSource. <http://www.teasource.com/teas/PreparingMatchaGreenTea.html>

Singh, Dr. Jagdev. "Herbal Tea Preparation Methods and List of Herbal Teas." Ayur Times. <https://www.ayurtimes.com/herbal-tea-preparation-methods-list-of-herbal-teas/>

"Tea: 6 Brilliant Effects on the Brain." PsyBlog. <http://www.spring.org.uk/2013/11/tea-6-brilliant-effects-on-the-brain.php>

"Tea – A Brief History of the Nation's Favourite Beverage." UK Tea and Infusions Association. <http://www.tea.co.uk/tea-a-brief-history>

"Tea and Diabetes." Diabetes.co.uk. <http://www.diabetes.co.uk/food/tea-and-diabetes.html>

"Tea Benefits: Weight Loss, Improved Bone Health and Mood." Medical News Today. <http://www.medicalnewstoday.com/articles/268509.php>

"The History of Tea." Teavana. <http://www.teavana.com/tea-info/history-of-tea>

"Top 10 London Tea Suppliers." About Travel. <http://golondon.about.com/od/londonteasuppliers/tp/London-Tea-Suppliers.htm>

"What is Inflammation? What Causes Inflammation?" Medical News Today.

<http://www.medicalnewstoday.com/articles/248423.php#acute_and_chronic_inflammation_compared>

"Where Can I Buy Better Tea?" LifeHacker.
<http://lifehacker.com/where-can-i-buy-better-tea-1619090729>

Zanteson, Lori. "Tea's Good for the Heart – Studies Show a Few Cups a Day Keep Heart Disease at Bay." Today's Dietician.
<http://www.todaysdietitian.com/newarchives/030413p18.shtml>

Image Credits

Cover Page Photo By Pixabay user Unsplash.

Page 1 Photo By Pixabay user Stevepb.

Page 3 Photo By Pixabay user Highnesser.

Page 6 Photo By Christophe Menebouef via Wikimedia Commons.

Page 9 Photo By Selena N.B.H. via Wikimedia Commons.

Page 13 Photo By Pixabay user Jill111.

Page 14 Photo By Patrick George via Wikimedia Commons.

Page 17 Photo By Mendhak via Wikimedia Commons.

Page 21 Photo By Saad Akhtar.

Page 26 Photo By Joekoz451 via Wikimedia Commons.

Page 28 Photo By Flickr user Bearepresa.

Page 32 Photo By Andre Karwath via Wikimedia Commons.

Page 35 Photo By Pixabay user Sadjack.

Page 38 Photo from FreeDigitalPhotos.net

Page 41 Photo Purchased from BigStockPhoto.com

Page 44 Photo Purchased from BigStockPhoto.com

Page 48 Photo By Pixabay user Nile.

Page 49 Photo By USAGI-WRP via Wikimedia Commons.

Page 52 Photo By Selena NBH via Wikimedia Commons.

Page 54 Photo By Flickr user Mr. Wabu.

Page 55 Photo By Pixabay user Dandelion L.

Page 59 Photo By USAGI-WRP via Wikimedia Commons.

Page 61 Photo By Kris Krug via Wikimedia Commons.

Page 64 Photo By Flickr user Aramek.

Page 67 Photo By Selena NBH via Wikimedia Commons

Page 71 Photo By Pixabay user Body-n-Care.

Page 75 Photo By Stinkie Pinkie via Wikimedia Commons.

Page 79 Photo By Revolution_Ferg via Wikimedia Commons.

Page 84 Photo By Avriette via Wikimedia Commons.

Page 87 Photo By Stan Shebs via Wikimedia Commons.

Page 90 Photo By MHM55 via Wikimedia Commons.

Page 94 Photo By Flickr user Kate.Fisher.

Page 97 Photo By Pixabay user PublicDomainPictures.

Page 100 Photo By Haneburger via Wikimedia Commons.

Page 105 Photo By Colin Smith via Wikimedia Commons.

Page 107 Photo By Pixabay user Unsplash.

Index

A

adulteration · 9, 10
Almond Tea · 56, 60
Alzheimer's · 37, 41, 51, 89
anti-inflammatory · 40, 45, 71, 81, 83, 85, 89, 92, 95, 107
antioxidants · 2, 35, 36, 50, 63, 65, 72, 77, 78, 83, 86, 87, 107
anxiety · 42, 74, 78, 80, 87, 93
Apple · 91, 92
aroma · 3, 2, 14, 16, 18, 21, 22, 29, 48, 52, 60, 65, 68, 76, 93, 94, 95, 96
arthritis · 39, 51, 57, 65, 72, 73, 76, 77, 83, 86, 95
Assam · 11, 56, 57, 59, 115
autoimmune · 39, 40

B

bancha · 15
Barley Tea · 69, 70
Black Currant Tea · 69, 92
black tea · 18, 19, 29, 43, 52, 56, 57, 58, 60, 61, 62, 85, 91, 92, 93, 95, 96, 103
blood pressure · 44, 63, 76, 79, 82
blooming tea · 30
blossoming tea · 30
Blueberry · 91, 92

C

caffeine · 38, 58, 63, 68

Calendula Tea · 69, 70
Camellia sinensis · 1, 4, 48, 49, 50, 55, 59, 60, 62, 64, 68, 90
cancer · 3, 2, 36, 37, 40, 50, 57, 65, 66, 71, 75, 76, 77, 86, 87, 89, 96
cardiovascular disease · 35, 44, 63, 70, 71, 72, 77, 86, 89, 107
Catnip · 69, 70
Ceylon · 56, 57, 60
Chaga · 69, 71
chai · 28, 29, 56, 61
chamomile · 1, 72, 74
Chamomile · 69, 72
China · 3, 4, 5, 7, 8, 11, 26, 29, 49, 52, 53, 55, 62, 64, 65, 67, 76, 77, 115
cholesterol · 44, 50, 51
Chrysanthemum · 69, 93, 113
Cinnamon · 69, 72
Coca · 69, 73
cold brewed · 31
Comfrey · 69, 73
Corn Silk · 69, 73
Cranberry · 91, 93

D

Damiana · 69, 74
Dandelion · 69, 74, 75, 115
Darjeeling · 56, 60
dark tea · 28, 29
diabetes · 35, 36, 37, 39, 43, 44, 71, 72, 107, 110
diseases · 3, 2, 37, 40, 41

E

East India Trading Company · 8, 11
Echinacea · 69, 74
endurance · 36

F

Fennel · 69, 75
Fenugreek · 69, 76, 82
flavor · 3, 2, 14, 15, 16, 18, 21, 22, 29, 31, 32, 33, 52, 54, 55, 56, 59, 60, 68, 73, 74, 76, 78, 81, 85, 93, 95
Floral teas · 90
flower tea · 30
flowering tea · 28, 30
fruit · 1, 82, 86, 90, 92, 93, 116
fruit teas · 90, 93

G

Ginger · 69, 76
Gingko Biloba · 69, 77
Ginseng · 69, 77
gongfu · 26
Graviola · 69, 77, 78
green tea · 14, 15, 26, 31, 36, 37, 38, 43, 44, 50, 51, 53, 56, 62, 63, 73, 103
gyokuro · 15, 16, 18, 31

H

health benefits · 3, 2, 11, 12, 35, 36, 43, 50, 52, 63, 68, 70, 76, 88, 107
herbal · 1, 3, 19, 25, 48, 67, 68, 71, 72, 73, 74, 75, 76, 77, 78, 80, 82, 83, 84, 85, 86, 87, 88, 89, 90, 92, 93, 95, 103, 109, 112
herbal decoction · 25
herbs · 1, 25, 26, 61, 67
Hibiscus · 69, 78, 79, 116
history · 3, 2, 3, 68, 110
hojicha · 15, 18
Holy Basil · 69, 78
Honeybush · 69, 78
Horsetail · 69, 79

I

iced tea · 28, 30, 31
immune · 40, 57, 72, 74, 77, 81, 83, 92, 95
inflammation · 39, 40, 43, 70, 73, 81, 82, 94, 111
infusion · 1, 4, 15, 16, 18, 25, 67, 70, 93

J

Jasmine Tea · 50, 52, 54

K

Kava · 69, 80
King Charles II · 8

L

Lavender · 91, 93, 94
leaves · 1, 4, 10, 13, 14, 18, 19, 20, 23, 24, 29, 30, 53, 54, 56, 64, 65, 68, 70, 73, 74, 78, 81, 82, 85, 86, 88, 89, 92, 99
Lemon Balm · 69, 80
Liquorice/licorice · 69, 80, 81
Linden · 91, 94
Lonjing · 50, 53
loose leaf · 22, 24, 27, 30, 32, 33, 97, 103, 105

M

masala · 29, 61
Masala Tea · 56, 61
matcha · 28, 31, 53
Matcha · 31, 50, 53, 109
memory · 42
Mint · 69, 81
Moringa · 69, 81
Mother's Milk · 69, 82
Mulberry · 69, 82
Mullein · 69, 82

N

Nettle · 69, 83

O

online · 97, 98, 99, 100, 102, 105

oolong tea · 43, 48, 56, 64, 65, 66
osteoporosis · 51, 57, 65, 86, 96

P

Parkinson's · 37, 41, 51
Parsley · 69, 83
Peach · 91, 95
Pineapple · 91, 95
polyphenols · 2, 35, 38, 43, 44, 57, 65, 87, 96
Poppy Seed · 69, 83, 84
preparation · 3, 2, 3, 13, 22, 23, 28, 109

R

Raspberry · 69, 84
Red Bush · 69, 85
Red Clover · 69, 85
rooibos · 1, 78, 85, 92, 103
Rooibos · 69, 85
Rose · 91, 95
rosehip · 1
Rosehip · 69, 86

S

Saffron · 69, 86
Sage · 69, 86, 87
Sassafras · 69, 88
sencha · 15, 16, 18
Sencha · 15, 50, 54

Senna · 69, 87, 117
smuggling · 9, 10
steeping · 1, 14, 20, 22, 78, 95
strainer · 18, 24
stroke · 45, 50, 57, 72
supplier · 98, 100

T

taxation · 8, 9, 10, 11
tea bags · 12, 13, 23, 30, 32, 33, 34, 61, 92, 97, 102
Tea caddy · 17
Tea cups · 17
tea house · 105
Tea infuser · 18
tea leaves · 14, 18, 19, 20, 23, 24, 99
Tea scoop · 18
tea shop · 48, 98, 105, 106
Teapot · 17, 18, 113
temperature · 14, 15, 16, 22, 24
theanine · 41, 42, 53, 57, 66
Tulsi · 69, 78, 88
Turmeric · 69, 88
types · 3, 2, 3, 13, 15, 16, 19, 21, 22, 28, 32, 33, 36, 37, 39, 40, 43, 48, 57, 66, 89, 95, 107, 108

V

Vanilla · 91, 96

W

water · 3, 1, 3, 4, 13, 14, 15, 16, 20, 22, 23, 24, 25, 26, 27, 29, 30, 31, 32, 49, 53, 54, 67, 74, 78, 83, 90, 93, 95, 107
white tea · 62, 63

Y

Yarrow · 69, 89
Yixing pot · 26

CPSIA information can be obtained
at www.ICGtesting.com
Printed in the USA
BVOW11s2247100118
504937BV00007B/71/P

9 780993 027826